T0311661

A VIDEO TEXTBOOK OF
GLUED IOLs

A VIDEO TEXTBOOK OF GLUED IOLs

Amar Agarwal, MS, FRCS, FRCOphth
Chairman and Managing Director
Dr. Agarwal's Group of Eye Hospitals and Eye Research Centre
Chennai, India

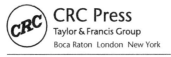

CRC Press
Taylor & Francis Group
Boca Raton London New York

CRC Press is an imprint of the
Taylor & Francis Group, an **informa** business

First published 2016 by SLACK Incorporated

Published 2024 by CRC Press
2385 NW Executive Center Drive, Suite 320, Boca Raton FL 33431

and by CRC Press
4 Park Square, Milton Park, Abingdon, Oxon, OX14 4RN

CRC Press is an imprint of Taylor & Francis Group, LLC

ISBN: 9781630912246 (pbk)
ISBN: 9781003526872 (ebk)

DOI: 10.1201/9781003526872

Additional resources can be found at
https://www.routledge.com/9781630912246

DEDICATION

This book is dedicated to a great surgeon and human being,
Terry Kim

BOOK CONTENTS

VIDEO CONTENT

All Videos Are From Dr. Agarwal's Eye Hospital

Acknowledgments

Nothing in this world moves without HIM and so also this book was only written by HIM.

ABOUT THE AUTHOR

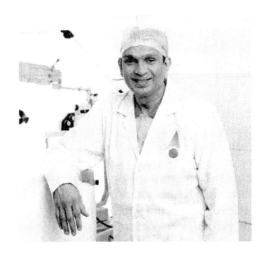

Amar Agarwal, MS, FRCS, FRCOphth, pioneered phakonit, which is phako with needle incision technology. This technique was popularized as bimanual phaco, microincision cataract surgery, or microphaco. He was the first to remove cataracts through a 0.7-mm tip with the technique called microphakonit. He also discovered no-anesthesia cataract surgery as well as FAVIT, a new technique for removing dropped nuclei. The air pump, which was a simple idea of using an aquarium fish pump to increase the fluid in the eye in bimanual phaco and coaxial phaco, has helped prevent surge, which became the basis for various techniques that involve forced infusion for small incision cataract surgery.

Dr. Agarwal also discovered a new refractive error called aberropia. He was the first to perform a combined surgery of microphakonit (700-micron cataract surgery) and a 25-gauge vitrectomy in the same patient, thus using the smallest incisions possible for cataract surgery and vitrectomy. He was also the first surgeon to implant a new mirror telescopic intraocular lens (IOL), the Lipshitz macular implant, for patients suffering from age-related macular degeneration.

Dr. Agarwal was the first in the world to implant a glued IOL, in which a posterior chamber IOL is fixed in an eye without any capsules using fibrin glue. The Malyugin ring for small-pupil cataract surgery was also modified as the Agarwal modification of the Malyugin ring for miotic pupil cataract surgeries with posterior capsular defects. Dr. Agarwal's Eye Hospital performed the first anterior segment transplantation in a 4-month-old child with anterior staphyloma. He also pioneered the technique of IOL scaffold, in which a 3-piece IOL is injected into an eye between the iris and the nucleus to prevent the nucleus from falling down in posterior capsular ruptures. Dr. Agarwal combined glued IOL and IOL scaffold in cases of posterior chamber rupture, in which there is no iris or capsular support, and termed the technique *glued IOL scaffold*. Doctors at Dr. Agarwal's Eye Hospital also performed the first glued endocapsular ring in a case of subluxated cataract.

Pre-Descemet's endothelial keratoplasty (PDEK) was created by Dr. Agarwal. In this technique, the pre–Descemet's layer and Descemet's membrane with endothelium are transplanted en bloc in patients with a diseased endothelium. Doctors at Dr. Agarwal's Eye Hospital performed the first contact lens-assisted collagen crosslinking (CACXL), a new technique for crosslinking thin corneas. He has also worked on E-DMEK, in which an endoilluminator is used to assist in DMEK surgeries. Dr. Agarwal designed a new instrument called the *trocar anterior chamber maintainer*, which helps provide infusion through the anterior chamber and works like a trocar cannula.

Dr. Agarwal has performed more than 150 live surgeries at various conferences. His videos have won many awards at the film festivals of the American Society of Cataract and Refractive Surgery, the American Academy of Ophthalmology, and the European Society of Cataract and Refractive Surgeons. He has also written more than 60 books, which have been published in various languages, including English, Spanish, and Polish. He also trains doctors from all over the world on phaco, bimanual phaco, LASIK surgery, and retinal surgery. He is Chairman and Managing Director of Dr. Agarwal's Group of Eye Hospitals, which has 60 eye hospitals all over the world.

CONTRIBUTING AUTHORS

Ashvin Agarwal, MS (Chapter 2)
Dr. Agarwal's Group of Eye Hospitals and Eye Research Centre
Chennai, India

Athiya Agarwal, MD, DO (Chapter 1)
Dr. Agarwal's Group of Eye Hospitals and Eye Research Centre
Chennai, India

Soosan Jacob, MS, FRCS, Dip NB (Chapter 4)
Dr. Agarwal's Group of Eye Hospitals and Eye Research Centre
Chennai, India

Vishal Jhanji, MD (Chapter 1)
Department of Ophthalmology and Visual Sciences
The Chinese University of Hong Kong
Hong Kong

Dhivya Ashok Kumar, MD (Chapter 5)
Dr. Agarwal's Group of Eye Hospitals and Eye Research Centre
Chennai, India

Priya Narang, MS (Chapter 3)
Narang Eye Hospital
Ahmedabad, India

PREFACE

This book is based on a simple yet powerful observation that all ophthalmologists across the globe are indebted to our patients for their faith in us. In complicated cataract cases, secondary IOL fixation is often necessary to optimize the visual outcome. This book will furnish all of the essential instructions for handling these complicated cases.

Although every surgeon will face a learning curve, I feel that paying attention to the minute details that we present in this book will enable the surgeon to rectify mistakes and benefit the patient.

The main goal of writing this book is to reveal the structured, accurate approach that results from many years of facilitating, researching, and teaching. Another aim is to provide readers with the most comprehensive and current information on glued fixation, and we hope that this book captures the current state of this vital and dynamic science from an international perspective.

In this book, I present some improvements and modifications to glued IOL surgery, as well as a few procedures combined with the glued IOL technique. The unifying thread in all the chapters is handling complications effectively. This book is published in the hope that it will interest all ophthalmologists and that it will offer effective solutions to problems that may arise.

I am greatly indebted to Dr. Maggi and Dr. Scharioth for being the pioneers in intrascleral fixation of intraocular lens and for showing us a path that future generations will always remember. I hope that this book helps readers to enhance visual outcomes for their patients.

—*Amar Agarwal, MS, FRCS, FRCOphth*

FOREWORD

Writing a foreword for this textbook, and accompanying videos, is a sweet pleasure. Dr. Amar Agarwal is an acknowledged leader in cataract surgery and its complications. He is widely known for his skill in repairing difficult surgical scenarios; he is equally skilled in preventing problems with his keen powers of observation and teaching surgeons how to manage complications with grace under pressure, turning challenges headed towards disaster into "saves."

Chapter 1 is a highly useful review of current cataract surgery, emphasizing the "handshake" maneuvers in bimanual cataract surgery. This chapter features the keystone on which all of the other maneuvers rest. The reader will be well served by reading this lengthy chapter several times and by carefully integrating the video footage into his or her surgical armamentarium.

Chapter 2 emphasizes the utility of intraocular glue to stabilize IOLs into the sclera. These techniques are key components that help in creating long-term solutions from unstable initial presentations.

Chapter 3 delves into the specific problems of posterior capsule defects and initially unstable nuclear fragments.

Chapter 4 segues into corneal stability in the course of advanced transplant maneuvers.

Chapter 5 completes the triad of glued IOL and implant stabilization.

Dr. Agarwal and his coauthors are to be congratulated on this extremely timely book that combines video, text, and accompanying illustrations into a powerful resource on the latest techniques in cataract surgery and complications. This treatise is a "must have" in the library of any cataract surgeon who aspires to be a master in cataract surgery.

—Roger Steinert, MD
Irving H. Leopold Professor and Chair of Ophthalmology
Director, Gavin Herbert Eye Institute
Professor of Biomedical Engineering
University of California, Irvine
Irvine, California

1

Indications, Surgical Procedure, and Mastering the Handshake Technique

Athiya Agarwal, MD, DO;
Amar Agarwal, MS, FRCS, FRCOphth;
and Vishal Jhanji, MD

Maggi and Maggi[1] were the first to report sutureless scleral fixation of a special intraocular lens (IOL) in 1997. In 2006, Gabor and Pavilidis[2] reported the scleral tuck and intrascleral haptic fixation of a posterior chamber IOL. Glued IOL, otherwise known as glued intrascleral haptic fixation of a PC IOL, is a technique for performing IOL implantation in eyes with absent or insufficient capsule support that was first described by the authors in 2007.[3] With this technique, they created scleral flaps and performed the haptic externalization under the scleral flaps, subsequently tucking the haptics into the intrascleral (Scharioth) tunnels and finally sealing with fibrin glue.[4-11]

The handshake technique[12] is a modification in which the IOL haptic is bimanually transferred from one glued IOL forceps to another under direct visualization in the pupillary plane until the tip of the haptic is grasped to facilitate easy externalization. It is crucial to grab the haptic with the glued

Agarwal A, ed.
A Video Textbook of Glued IOLs (pp 1-36).
© 2016 Taylor & Francis Group.

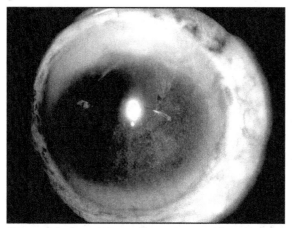

Figure 1-1. Posterior capsular rupture with subluxated endocapsular ring. (Reprinted with permission from Dr. Agarwal's Eye Hospital.)

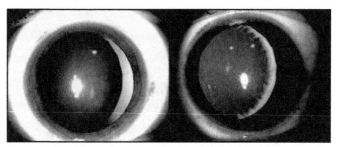

Figure 1-2. Subluxated cataract. (Reprinted with permission from Dr. Agarwal's Eye Hospital.)

IOL forceps from the tip and not from anywhere else down the entire length of the haptic. The glued IOL technique has grown in popularity with so many pioneers modifying the technique.[13-17]

Long-term studies on glued IOL with complications showing IOL tilt and the slow movement capture of the glued IOL on video have all been published.[18-25]

INDICATIONS

The glued IOL technique can be used in cases of posterior capsular rupture (Figure 1-1), subluxated IOL, cataract (Figure 1-2), or coloboma of the lens.

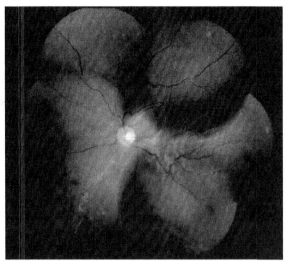

Figure 1-3. Retinal detachment. (Reprinted with permission from Dr. Agarwal's Eye Hospital.)

PREOPERATIVE EVALUATION

Preoperative evaluation of any patient undergoing this surgery is a must because these eyes may have had previous surgery (Figure 1-3). The postoperative outcome of this surgery depends on the proper preoperative evaluation of the case. Often, these eyes are associated with an element of vitritis and cystoid macular edema (Figure 1-4) or may be associated with corneal decompensation after an eventful phacoemulsification surgery. The role of preoperative evaluation cannot be underestimated because it helps to explain the visual prognosis to the patient. Fundus examination is an integral part of the routine ophthalmic examination and should always be done. Indirect ophthalmoscopy is a useful technique for providing a wide-angle view of the fundus, screening for retinal disease, and examining the peripheral retina.

LENS

The lenticular assessment is extremely important in cases of traumatic subluxation or dislocation. In subluxation, the edge of the lens might be visible in the pupil. In complete dislocation (luxation), the lens displaces into the vitreous or, rarely, into the anterior chamber.

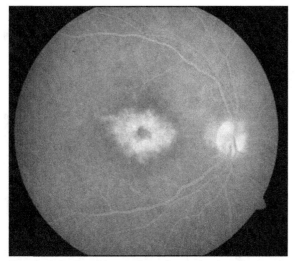

Figure 1-4. Cystoid macular edema: fundus fluorescein angiography showing flower petal appearance. (Reprinted with permission from Dr. Agarwal's Eye Hospital.)

WHITE-TO-WHITE DIAMETER

The corneal white-to-white (WTW) diameter should always be measured. If the horizontal WTW diameter is approximately 11 mm, then a horizontal glued IOL procedure can be done, which means the flaps can be made at the 3 o'clock and 9 o'clock positions. If the WTW diameter is more than 11 mm, it would be better to do a vertical glued IOL, which means the scleral flaps are made at the 12 o'clock and 6 o'clock positions (Figure 1-5). This is performed because the vertical cornea will always be shorter than the horizontal cornea, so there will be more haptic to tuck and glue (Figure 1-6). This idea was suggested by Dr. Jeevan Ladi.[26]

FIBRIN GLUE

Tissue adhesives can be categorized into 1 of 2 main classes—synthetic (eg, cyanoacrylate- and acrylic-based polymers) or biological (eg, fibrin glue and biodendrimers).[27] The sealer protein generally has 2 major components (fibrinogen and thrombin) and 2 coagulating factors (aprotinin [fibrinolysis inhibitor] and calcium chloride). The setting time of the mixture is usually dependent on the thrombin concentration. A fast-setting mixture sets

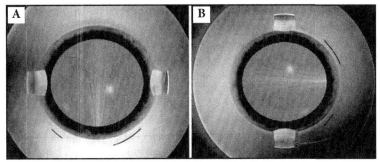

Figure 1-5. (A). Horizontal glued IOL. Note the smaller amount of haptic available to tuck and glue. (B) Vertical glued IOL. Note the larger amount of haptic available to tuck and glue. (Reprinted with permission from Dr. Agarwal's Eye Hospital.)

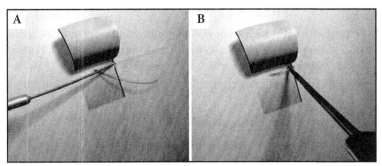

Figure 1-6. Scharioth intrascleral pocket and haptic tuck. (A) Intrascleral pocket created with a 26-gauge needle. (B) Haptic of the PC IOL tucked in the intrascleral pocket. (Reprinted with permission from Dr. Agarwal's Eye Hospital.)

within 30 seconds, and a slow-setting mixture sets within 1 to 2 minutes. Fibrin glue is designed to mimic the last stage of blood coagulation. Factor XIIIa is a transglutaminase that catalyzes the final steps in the formation of a fibrin clot. The enzyme stabilizes the fibrin clot through crosslinking (CXL) of fibrin monomers to each other, as well as CXL of fibronectin and a 2-plasmin inhibitor to fibrin. Fibrin glue clot formation starts with the activation of factor XIII by thrombin. The activated factor XIII then hydrolyzes prothrombin to thrombin. Thrombin converts fibrinogen into fibrin. Fibrin self-assembles into fibers to form a 3-dimensional matrix. Thrombin also activates factor XIIIa (present in the fibrinogen component of the glue), which stabilizes the clot by CXL of fibrin fibers and by inducing polymerization of the fibers in the presence of calcium ions. The main disadvantages of fibrin glue include long preparation time for thrombin-induced activation of the enzyme, proteolytic degradation, and low adhesion strength.

Also, there is a latent risk of viral transmission, although various strategies have been developed to reduce this risk.

Commercially Available Fibrin Glue

Fibrin glue was developed in 1972 by Matras et al.[28] Fibrin sealant has been available in Europe since 1978, and blood bank- or laboratory-derived fibrin sealants have been used in the United States since the 1980s. Tisseel (Baxter) was the first fibrin sealant approved by the United States Food and Drug Administration (FDA). Fibrin sealant is now approved by the FDA for use as a topical hemostat, sealant, and adhesive. All fibrin sealants in use have 2 major ingredients—purified fibrinogen and purified thrombin derived from human or bovine blood. Many sealants have 2 additional ingredients—human blood factor XIII and aprotinin, which is derived from cows' lungs.

There are currently 5 FDA-approved commercial fibrin sealants distributed by US companies: Tisseel (Baxter), Artiss (Baxter), Evicel (Johnson & Johnson), Cryoseal (Thermogenesis), and Vitagel (Orthovita).

- Tisseel, Artiss, and Evicel fibrin sealants are prepared from human pooled plasma.
- Cryoseal is prepared from individual units of plasma.
- Vitagel is prepared from individual units of plasma, bovine collagen, and bovine thrombin.

In Europe, Tisseel/Tissucol, Beriplast (Aventis Behring), and Quixil (Johnson & Johnson Wound Management/Omrix Biopharmaceuticals) are approved for use. Tisseel and Beriplast both use aprotinin (fibrinolysis inhibitor) derived from bovine sources. Quixil uses a synthetic fibrinolysis inhibitor (tranexamic acid) to eliminate the risk of immunologic response. In India, ReliSeal (Reliance Life Sciences) is commercially available.

Application Techniques

The 2 components of fibrin glue—fibrinogen and thrombin—can be applied either simultaneously or sequentially, depending on the physician's preference. When simultaneous application is preferred, both the components are loaded into 2 syringes with tips forming a common port (eg, Duploject syringe [Baxter]). When injected, the 2 components are mixed in equal volumes at the point of delivery. The setting time depends on the concentration of the thrombin component. For sequential application, thrombin is first applied to the area of interest, followed by a thin layer of fibrinogen. When apposition is required between 2 surfaces, thrombin solution may be applied to one and fibrinogen to the other surface. We prefer to keep 2 separate syringes because they are easier to use.

INSTRUMENTS

The following instruments are required for the procedure:

1. One-toothed forceps

2. Tying forceps (at least 3 for the surgeon and 1 for the assistant)

3. Corneal scissors

4. Stab knife

5. Keratome blades

6. Scleral flap dissector

7. A 20- or 22-gauge scleral needle to make a sclerotomy 1 mm behind the limbus under the flaps (a microvitreoretinal [MVR] blade can be used, but a needle attached to a syringe is easier)

8. Trocar infusion cannula, or a trocar anterior chamber (AC) maintainer

9. Twenty-three–gauge glued IOL forceps (need 2 for handshake technique)

10. One 26-gauge needle that can be bent to create the Scharioth tunnels (can use 25 or 27 gauge if 26 gauge is not available)

11. Fibrin glue

CONJUNCTIVAL PERITOMY

If a manual non-phaco technique or a nonfoldable glued IOL implantation is being performed, it is better to have the superior rectus secured because exposure is better. In such cases, prepare the conjunctival peritomy in the areas where the scleral flaps will be made. Adequate, but not excessive, cautery should be done to stop any bleeding vessels.

SCLERAL MARKING

It is imperative that the scleral flaps be 180 degrees apart; if not, the IOL will be decentered. For this reason, it is better to use a scleral marker, which creates marks on the cornea to verify that the scleral flaps created are diagonally opposite (Figure 1-7).

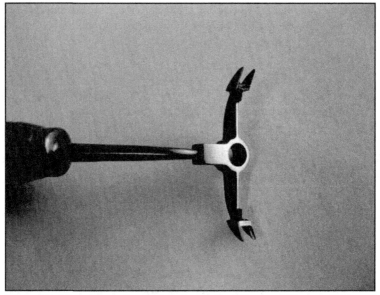

Figure 1-7. Ashvin Agarwal's scleral marker (Epsilon). The special feature of this tool is that it makes marks for the scleral flaps. It also measures 11 mm, so it is immediately apparent if the WTW diameter is too large. (Reprinted with permission from Dr. Agarwal's Eye Hospital.)

SCLERAL FLAP PREPARATION

The flaps should be 2.5 × 2.5 mm with the base at the limbus. A flap that is too large is not ideal because the haptic has to traverse a longer distance to get tucked. There are many ways in which the scleral flap can be prepared, similar to how a trabeculectomy flap is prepared. At times, it is cumbersome to create these flaps when using the nondominant hand. A simple way to create the scleral flaps (Figure 1-8) is to first use a knife to make a mark on the sclera to up to half-thickness (see Figure 1-8A), being careful not to make it too deep or too shallow. Once the marks are made, take the hockey-flap dissector (the same one used to make a scleral tunnel) and pass it from one end of the flap (see Figure 1-8B) until it comes out the other end (see Figure 1-8C). Then, move the dissector outward so that the flap is created. The flap is then lifted (see Figure 1-8D), and any bleeding vessels can be cauterized.

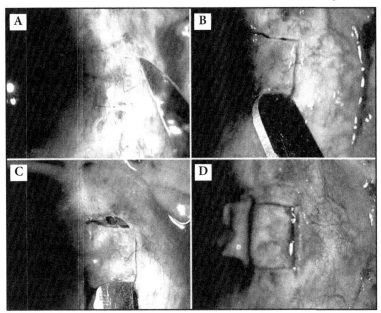

Figure 1-8. Scleral flap creation. (A) The knife first makes half-thickness marks. (B) The dissector passes from one end of the flap. (C) The dissector comes out from the other end. (D) The dissector is moved outward to complete the flap, and the flap is lifted and checked. (Reprinted with permission from Dr. Agarwal's Eye Hospital.)

INFUSION WITH A TROCAR CANNULA

Infusion of fluid into the eye can be done by using a sutureless 23/25-gauge trocar cannula (Figure 1-9). The advantage is that there is no disruption of conjunctival integrity, no need for suturing the sclerotomy, and a reduction in surgical time. Insertion and removal of the cannula are faster than with a conventional 20-gauge infusion cannula. The trocar infusion kit is available separately and can be used by anterior segment surgeons in special situations. It contains a scleral guide, an inserter, and an infusion cannula. The scleral guide is inserted into the pars plana approximately 3.0 mm from the limbus with the help of the inserter (see Figures 1-9A and B), the inserter is removed, and the infusion cannula connected to the infusion bottle is then inserted (see Figures 1-9C and D). During removal of the cannula, the infusion is switched off and the scleral guide removed. No suture is applied in the sclerotomy site. We noted that the surgical time needed to fixate the infusion cannula was reduced when 23-gauge infusion was used. It was also safe and easy in the hands of anterior segment surgeons because the trocar

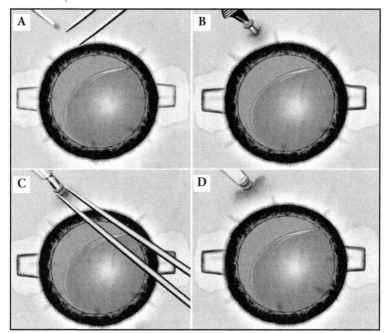

Figure 1-9. Insertion of 23-gauge trocar and cannula for glued IOL surgery. (A) A 23-gauge trocar is placed 3.0 mm from the limbus. The distance is measured using a caliper. (B) The trocar is inserted into the pars plana. (C,D) The inserter is removed and an infusion cannula connected to the infusion bottle is inserted. (Reprinted with permission from Agarwal A, Jacob S. *Illustrative Guide to Cataract Surgery: A Step-by-Step Approach to Refining Surgical Skills.* Thorofare, NJ: SLACK Incorporated; 2011.)

is inserted and the infusion cannula is fixated. Always ensure that the tip of the infusion cannula is in the vitreous cavity before the infusion is started. If the pupil is miotic, an iris retractor can be used to retract the iris and check that the infusion cannula is in the vitreous cavity. Direct visualization of the cannula during entrance and exit decreases the risk for complications.

Fixating a normal 20-gauge infusion cannula requires time to cut the conjunctiva, perform cautery, and then suture the infusion cannula to the sclera. Compared with the 20-gauge infusion cannula, the 23-gauge cannula caused significantly less postoperative pain and discomfort. If a 23-gauge trocar cannula kit is readily available in the operating room, it would be simple to use in glued IOL implantation by the anterior segment surgeon.

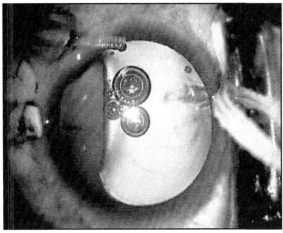

Figure 1-10. AC maintainer. Note the coloboma of the lens. In such cases, we perform lensectomy vitrectomy with glued IOL implantation. (Reprinted with permission from Dr. Agarwal's Eye Hospital.)

INFUSION WITH AN ANTERIOR CHAMBER MAINTAINER

Another alternative is to fix an AC maintainer in the eye. For this procedure, a clear corneal incision with a sideport knife should be made and then the AC maintainer passed in the eye. It should be parallel to the iris and in an area that does not affect the surgical view (Figure 1-10).

TROCAR CANNULA VS ANTERIOR CHAMBER MAINTAINER

Infusion of fluid can be done with either a trocar cannula or an AC maintainer. The advantage of a trocar cannula is that it is in the vitreous cavity and does not hamper the surgical view. It also does not push back or touch the iris. The disadvantage is that an anterior segment surgeon might not have easy access to a trocar cannula, as would a posterior segment surgeon. The trocar cannula must be in the vitreous cavity before turning on the infusion so that the fluid does not go into the subretinal space. It may be difficult sometimes to visualize in small pupils.

The advantages of an AC maintainer are that it is easily available for an anterior segment surgeon, is reautoclavable, and there is no issue of having to be careful that the tip is in the subretinal space. The disadvantage of the AC maintainer is that the clear corneal incision does not always match the size of the AC maintainer accurately, which can lead to the AC maintainer coming out in the middle of surgery and having to be refixed. Another issue with the AC maintainer is that when the AC maintainer fluid is turned on, it pushes the iris back, creating a deep AC. When making the 20-gauge needle sclerotomy under the scleral flaps, it is possible to hit the iris root as the iris is pushed back by the fluid. A solution to this is to fix the AC maintainer, create the 20-gauge sclerotomies, and then turn on the infusion.

TROCAR ANTERIOR CHAMBER MAINTAINER

An AC maintainer may not match the knife entry. When we make a clear corneal incision, the entry can be too big or too small for the AC maintainer, which can lead to a fluid leak or difficulty in passing the AC maintainer into the eye. In vitreous surgery, a trocar cannula provides a tight and correct fit, but cannot be passed through clear corneal incisions because they can produce a wound gape.

We use the trocar cannula, but pass it through the sclera approximately 0.5 mm from the limbus and then direct it to the AC just above the iris. This way, we have a tunnel entry and are able to create a trocar AC maintainer (Figure 1-11) that does not damage the cornea and is also self-fixing. It can be removed by simply pulling it out, and the wound closes without a leak.

This is very helpful for the following reasons:

- Anterior segment surgeons may not want to go to the pars plana.
- It can be used for any case of posterior capsular rupture, sutured IOL, or glued IOL.
- The corneal surgeon can use it for unfolding an endothelial graft or a pre-Descemet's endothelial keratoplasty graft with air. It must be fixed and connected to an air pump to infuse continuous air in the AC.

All in all, a trocar AC maintainer (Mastel, USA) makes life easier for the surgeon because it provides the advantages of both the trocar cannula and the AC maintainer.

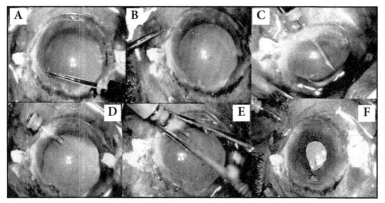

Figure 1-11. Trocar AC maintainer. (A) 25-gauge trocar. (B) The trocar enters the sclera 0.5 mm from the limbus and parallel to the limbus. (C) The trocar is turned and passed into the eye perpendicular to the limbus and enters the AC. (D) The trocar is removed and the cannula kept in place. (E) The intravenous set connected to the balanced salt solution bottle is now locked onto the cannula. (F) The trocar AC maintainer is removed at the end of surgery, and no leak is noted. (Reprinted with permission from Dr. Agarwal's Eye Hospital.)

INFUSION GAUGE

A 23-, 25-, or 27-gauge trocar cannula can be used for infusion. It is best to use a 25 gauge if available because the vitrectomy probes are 23 gauge, and so there will not be a collapse of the eye. For a trocar AC maintainer, a 25 gauge is ideal; a smaller one would need an air pump in the infusion (gas-forced infusion) that is not required otherwise. If a 25 gauge is not available, a 23 gauge can be substituted.

SCLERAL FLAPS OR INFUSION: WHICH COMES FIRST?

In the case of a patient posted for secondary IOL in aphakia or a fresh ectopia lentis, it is better to create the scleral flaps first because the globe is firm and it is easy to create the scleral flaps. In a case of a posterior capsular rupture in which the corneal or scleral tunnel is open and a glued IOL surgery will be performed, it is better to first fix the infusion because fluid is flowing inside the eye. The open wound can be sutured (either clear corneal or scleral tunnel), and then the infusion can be fixed for fluid so that the globe becomes firm. Then, it is easy to create the scleral flaps. Creating the

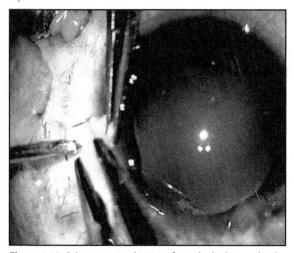

Figure 1-12. Sclerotomy made 1 mm from the limbus under the scleral flap using a 20-gauge needle. (Reprinted with permission from Dr. Agarwal's Eye Hospital.)

scleral flaps in eyes that are open is tricky because the eyeball is soft. Drs. Francis Price and Yuri McKee have designed a Mastel diamond knife for creating the scleral flaps.

SCLEROTOMIES UNDER THE FLAP

Two straight sclerotomies with a 20/22-gauge needle are made approximately 1.0 mm from the limbus under the existing scleral flaps (Figure 1-12). The sclerotomies should be directed obliquely into the midvitreous cavity so that the iris is not hit, which can happen if the sclerotomies are made in a horizontal direction. Twenty-three–gauge glued IOL forceps can be used to make a 20-gauge sclerotomy. If a 22-gauge needle is used for the sclerotomy, 23/25-gauge glued IOL forceps must be used for externalizing the haptics.

An MVR blade also may be used for creating the sclerotomies. We prefer a 20/22-gauge needle because it can be thrown away once the sclerotomies are made.

VITRECTOMY

Vitrectomy is performed using a 20/23/25-gauge vitrectomy probe. A good vitrectomy is crucial for preventing vitreous traction and chances of

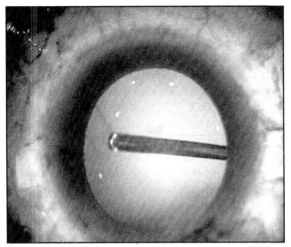

Figure 1-13. 23-gauge vitrectomy to remove anterior and midvitreous. (Reprinted with permission from Dr. Agarwal's Eye Hospital.)

retinal breaks and retinal detachments. A 23- or 25-gauge vitrectomy probe, such as those available with posterior vitrectomy machines or with phaco machines, can be passed through the sclerotomy under the scleral flap (Figure 1-13). When using the vitrectomy setup of a phaco machine, remember that those vitrectomy probes are sometimes 20-gauge and will not pass through a 20-gauge needle sclerotomy. In such a case, a clear corneal incision can be made (see Figure 1-12), and the vitrectomy may be performed through the clear corneal incision.

CORNEAL INCISIONS

Two corneal incisions must be made; one is the main corneal incision for the IOL implantation, and the other is the sideport through which the glued IOL forceps can pass for the handshake technique. Remember that the incisions should be 90 degrees to the scleral flaps and not parallel to them; otherwise, it is very difficult to perform the handshake technique.

IOL TYPES

The glued IOL procedure can be performed well with a rigid polymethylmethacrylate (PMMA) IOL, 3-piece PC IOL, or an IOL with modified PMMA haptics. Therefore, an entire inventory of sutured, sclera-fixated IOLs with eyelets is not needed. In dislocated PC PMMA IOL or 3-piece IOLs, the same IOL can be repositioned, thereby reducing the need for further manipulation. The one IOL that cannot be glued is the single-piece foldable IOL, because a firm haptic is required to tuck and glue.

It is best to use a 3-piece IOL because the haptics do not break, as do the single-piece nonfoldable IOLs. A foldable 3-piece IOL is even better because the incision does not need to be enlarged. The length of a regular, foldable 3-piece IOL is 13 mm. The 3-piece nonfoldable IOLs are 13.5 mm.

When using a 3-piece foldable IOL, any brand is good as long as it is 13 mm. The advantage of the Bausch + Lomb IOL is that the injector is very good. It has a plunger mechanism that enables the surgeon to use one hand to inject the IOL. The incision has to be enlarged a bit because the tip of the cartridge is a bit broader than those from other companies. If the incision is a bit larger, the cartridge tip can enter the AC easily. The Abbott Medical Optics IOL is very good because the haptics are very strong. If using a rotating mechanism injector, ask the assistant to rotate. The Alcon IOL is also good. Another IOL, popularized by Dr. Roger Steinert and later by Dr. Francis Price and Dr. Sadeer B. Hannush, is the Aaren EC3 PAL IOL, which is a 3-piece IOL with excellent haptic strength. On the nonfoldable IOL issue, a scleral tunnel of approximately 7 mm must be made. It is better not to make this a corneal incision. If a corneal incision is present, suture it, and after doing a conjunctival peritomy, make a scleral tunnel to implant the IOL. Always use a 3-piece nonfoldable IOL.

FOLDABLE IOL INJECTORS

It is preferable to use a plunger-type injector for better coordination, although a rotating mechanism-type injector may also be used. In the latter case, the assistant gently maneuvers the IOL forward as the surgeon holds the injector with one hand and the glued IOL forceps with the other hand. While introducing the injector, it is advisable to have the injector tip within the mouth of the incision and not use wound-assisted injection of the IOL, which can lead to a sudden uncontrolled entry of the IOL into the eye and a consequent IOL drop into the vitreous.

LUCKY 7 SIGN

In the glued IOL technique, the unfolding of an IOL with an appreciation of a "lucky 7" sign (a term coined by Dr. Thomas Oetting) for the leading

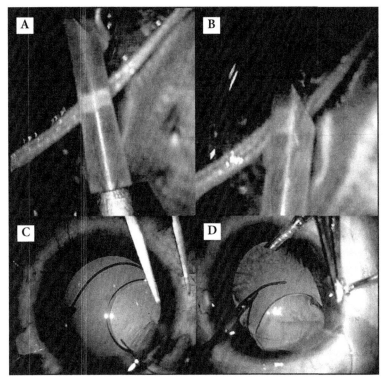

Figure 1-14. The lucky 7 sign in glued IOL surgery. (A, B) The lucky 7 sign for leading haptic: folding of the haptic in cartridge and an IOL dialer used to straighten it. The small, bent portion of the haptic should be slightly out of the cartridge, indicating the small portion of the 7. The rest of the haptic is straight and inside the cartridge, indicating the long portion of the 7. (C) An inverse C sign of the leading haptic and an upright C sign for the trailing haptic. (D) Reverse unfolding of an IOL. Note that the trailing haptic has an upright C pattern and the trailing haptic has an inverse C. (Reprinted with permission from Dr. Agarwal's Eye Hospital.)

haptic and a "C" sign for the trailing haptic is of utmost importance.[29] As the IOL is loaded, the surgeon ensures that the leading haptic extrudes from the cartridge in the form of the "lucky 7" (Figure 1-14A). The initial short portion of the 7 should be protruding to facilitate grasping by the glued IOL forceps, ensuring safe IOL unfolding and nullifying the chances of an IOL drop. The IOL is unfolded and the injector is withdrawn at the end so that the trailing haptic lies at the corneal incision. The trailing haptic showcases an "upright C" sign at this stage (Figure 1-14B). Any inability to decipher the lucky 7 sign or any variation, such as folding the haptic in the cartridge for the leading haptic, should be noted because any sudden, jerky, uncontrolled unfolding can lead to an IOL drop and the IOL injection should be withheld if possible. If folded in the cartridge, the haptic can be straightened out with an IOL dialer (Figure 1-14C), and a lucky 7 sign can be appreciated. If the IOL has already unfolded in a reverse fashion (Figure 1-14D), the IOL can be flipped upside down in the eye and the surgery continued. Appreciation of an upright C sign for the trailing haptic in the AC instead of at the corneal incision should be taken as a warning sign because slippage of the leading haptic at this juncture can lead to an IOL drop. The importance of "Z" and "S" signs has been highlighted for IOL unfolding because the angulation and geometry of the IOL result in different optical results and undesirable effective lens positions in the eye if inserted upside down. In glued IOL surgery, the horizon of error for IOL unfolding is negligible due to absence of posterior capsule. It is imperative to identify this problem at the beginning of an IOL injection. At this juncture, the appreciation of the lucky 7 sign comes into play because it is still possible to abort the IOL insertion, withdraw the injector, and load the IOL again.

LEADING HAPTIC EXTERNALIZATION

The externalization of the haptic of the IOL intraoperatively is the key step in glued IOL surgery. The important step is to grab the tip of the haptic with the end-opening forceps. If the surgeon grasps the haptic in some place other than the tip and tries to externalize it, the haptic may get deformed or break. This precise step of manipulation of an IOL haptic should be perfected in order to decrease the surgical time. This is made easier now with the handshake technique.

A 3-piece foldable IOL is loaded and the haptic is slightly protruded from the cartridge (Figure 1-15). The cartridge is entered into the AC and the glued IOL forceps is simultaneously introduced from the sclerotomy site to grasp the tip of the haptic. The IOL is then gradually injected into the eye. If the injector is a rotating mechanism, the assistant should rotate the injector. The haptic should not be externalized until the optic completely unfolds inside the eye; otherwise the optic can break. Once the optic is unfolded (Figure 1-16), the glued IOL forceps pull the haptic out and externalize it. The haptic can then be caught by an assistant.

When the surgeon injects the IOL, one hand is holding the tip of the haptic. There is no fear of the IOL falling into the vitreous cavity for 2 reasons:

1. The tip of the haptic is caught with the forceps, so the IOL cannot go down.

2. The trailing haptic is still outside the eye. If the forceps slip and the haptic is missed, the trailing haptic can still be caught and the IOL would not fall into the vitreous cavity.

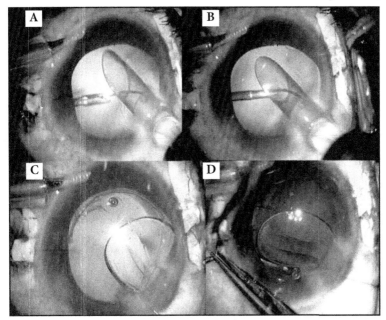

Figure 1-15. Leading haptic externalization in glued IOL. (A) IOL in injector. Note that the haptic tip is slightly out of the cartridge and the cartridge is in the AC. There is no wound-assisted injection. The glued IOL forceps (Epsilon) are passed through the sclerotomy with the other hand ready to grasp the tip of the haptic. Wound-assisted injection should not be done because the injection might happen too fast, which can either break the IOL or push it so fast that it might go into the vitreous cavity. (B) Tip of the haptic grasped with the glued IOL forceps. (C) Injection of the IOL continued. If it is a plunger-type injector, the surgeon can do it, but if it is a rotating-mechanism injector, an assistant can rotate the injector for release of the IOL because both hands of the surgeon are occupied. The IOL has unfolded inside the eye, and then only the cartridge is removed. Note that one hand is still holding the haptic tip but has not yet externalized the tip. If the haptic is externalized and the haptic before the IOL has unfolded from the cartridge, the IOL can break. (D) The haptic is externalized and the assistant tries to grasp the haptic so that it does not fall back inside the eye. (Reprinted with permission from Agarwal A, Jacob S, Kumar DA, Agarwal A, Narasimhan S, Agarwal A. Handshake technique for glued intrascleral haptic fixation of a posterior chamber intraocular lens. *J Cataract Refract Surg.* 2013;39[3]:317-322.)

TRAILING HAPTIC EXTERNALIZATION

The trailing haptic is caught with the first glued IOL forceps and flexed into the AC (Figure 1-17). The haptic is transferred from the first forceps to the second using the handshake technique (Figure 1-18). The second forceps are passed through the sideport. The first forceps are then passed through

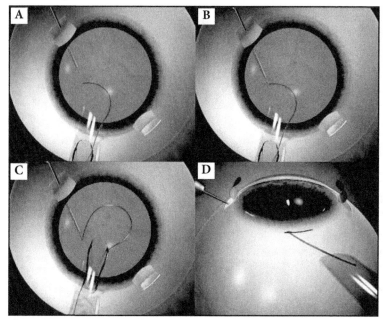

Figure 1-16. Illustration showing leading haptic externalization. (A) Haptic outside the cartridge and glued IOL forceps ready to grasp the haptic tip. (B) Haptic tip caught with the forceps. (C) Injection of the IOL is continued until the optic unfolds inside the AC. One should not externalize the haptic until the entire optic has unfolded; otherwise, the optic can break. (D) Haptic externalized. (Reprinted with permission from Agarwal A, Jacob S, Kumar DA, Agarwal A, Narasimhan S, Agarwal A. Handshake technique for glued intrascleral haptic fixation of a posterior chamber intraocular lens. *J Cataract Refract Surg.* 2013;39[3]:317-322.)

the sclerotomy under the scleral flap. The haptic is transferred from the second forceps back to the first using the handshake technique once again. The haptic tip is grasped with the first forceps, pulled toward the sclerotomy, and externalized.

HANDSHAKE TECHNIQUE

The handshake technique is particularly applicable in cases of slippage of the haptic during externalization or in cases of subluxation of 3-piece IOLs, in which the tip of the haptic can be easily approached by transferring the haptic between 2 glued IOL forceps. The handshake technique is a modification of the glued IOL procedure in which the IOL haptic is bimanually transferred from one end-opening forceps to another under direct visualization

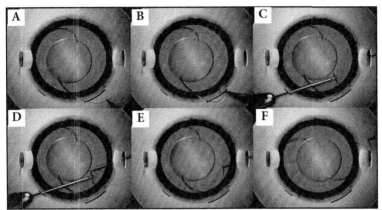

Figure 1-17. Handshake technique: illustration of trailing haptic externalization. (A) The trailing haptic is caught with the first glued IOL forceps. (B) Haptic flexed into the AC. (C) The haptic is transferred from the first forceps to the second using the handshake technique. The second forceps are passed through the sideport. (D) The first forceps are passed through the sclerotomy under the scleral flap. (E) The haptic is transferred from the second forceps back to the first using the handshake technique. (F) The haptic externalized. (Reprinted with permission from Agarwal A, Jacob S, Kumar DA, Agarwal A, Narasimhan S, Agarwal A. Handshake technique for glued intrascleral haptic fixation of a posterior chamber intraocular lens. *J Cataract Refract Surg.* 2013;39[3]:317-322.)

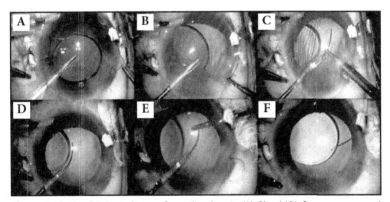

Figure 1-18. Handshake technique for trailing haptic. (A) Glued IOL forceps are passed through the sideport. (B) The trailing haptic grasped with forceps and flexed to make them enter the AC. (C) Trailing haptic passed into the AC and, with the handshake technique, the haptic grasp is shifted from one forceps to the other. Note the dimpling on the cornea as the main incision is open due to the forceps passage. (D) Trailing haptic caught with forceps passed through the sideport. Note no dimpling on the cornea because the main port incision is closed. It is now easy to see the tip of the haptic. (E) Glued IOL forceps passed through the sclerotomy and tip of the haptic grasped. Once again, the handshake technique helps pass the haptic from one forceps to the other. (F) The trailing haptic externalized. (Reprinted with permission from Agarwal A, Jacob S, Kumar DA, Agarwal A, Narasimhan S, Agarwal A. Handshake technique for glued intrascleral haptic fixation of a posterior chamber intraocular lens. *J Cataract Refract Surg.* 2013;39[3]:317-322.)

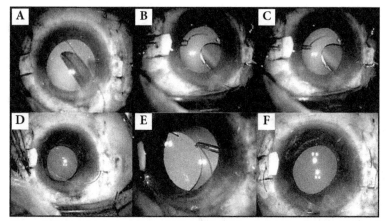

Figure 1-19. Handshake technique. (A) Foldable IOL haptic is below the iris. (B) Glued IOL forceps are passed through the opposite sclerotomy site while the other forceps are ready to receive the haptic. (C) The leading haptic is grasped with forceps, and the haptic tip is fed into another forceps. (D) One haptic is externalized, and an assistant holds the haptic. (E) Trailing haptic caught with the glued IOL forceps. (F) Both of the haptics are externalized under the scleral flaps. (Reprinted with permission from Agarwal A. Handshake technique for glued intrascleral haptic fixation of a posterior chamber intraocular lens. *J Cataract Refract Surg.* 2013;39[3]:317-322.)

in the pupillary plane, which is continued until the tip of the haptic is grasped so that it can be externalized easily.

The handshake technique can be used in a variety of situations. For example, it is essential to hold the haptic at its tip before exteriorizing it so that it does not snag on the sclerotomy while being brought out. The handshake transfer of the haptic between the 2 glued IOL forceps is continued until the tip of the haptic is caught by the forceps on the side to which the haptic is to be exteriorized. The handshake technique also can be used to regrasp the haptic if one of the haptics is not caught or if it gets released accidentally after grasping. The glued IOL forceps are introduced through the sideport, which becomes invaluable in this situation. The handshake technique involves 2 glued IOL forceps, one of which holds one haptic (Figure 1-19). The other glued IOL forceps are introduced into the eye and, the first hand then transfers the haptic into the second glued IOL forceps, such that the first hand now becomes free. This technique is especially useful for subluxated 3-piece IOLs because it enables easy intraocular maneuverability of the entire haptic or IOL within a closed-globe system. The glued IOL forceps are introduced through the sclerotomy to grasp the IOL while a vitrectomy is done all around the IOL to free vitreous traction. Once the IOL is free, glued IOL forceps are introduced through the other sclerotomy and the IOL is exchanged between hands until the tip of the haptic is grasped. The haptic is then exteriorized and held by the assistant while the handshake maneuver is used for the second haptic in a similar manner. This allows refixation of the same IOL with a closed-chamber approach with minimal intervention.

No-Assistant Technique

The "no-assistant" technique is an effort to decrease the dependence on an assistant[17] as well as to make the process of externalization of haptics, which is considered to be the most technically demanding part of the surgery, easier. The no-assistant technique was conceptualized by Dr. Priya Narang.

Three Hands in Glued IOL Surgery

In a standard glued IOL surgery, the assistant holds the leading haptic while the surgeon engages in the externalization of the trailing haptic. A level of surgical expertise is required for the assistant to hold the haptic properly. Undue pressure on the haptic causes it to flatten, which makes it difficult to tuck. Inability of the assistant to hold the leading haptic along the correct plane causes IOL torsion and renders the procedure difficult at times.

Physics

The entire technique works on a simple principle of physics—vector forces. The midpupillary plane is the major contributor to the success of this technique.

Standard Scenario vs the No-Assistant Technique

After externalization of the leading haptic, there is a tendency for it to slip back into the AC due to vector forces acting along the axis of the IOL. With the no-assistant technique, the trailing haptic crosses the midpupillary plane and, nearing the 6 o'clock position, the vector forces act in a way that causes further extrusion of the leading haptic from the sclerotomy site, with virtually no chance of slippage into the AC.

Surgical Technique

The trailing haptic is grasped with the glued IOL forceps while the left hand still holds onto the leading haptic. The trailing haptic is then moved

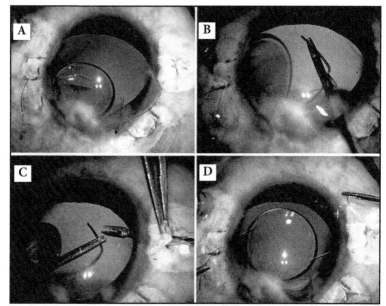

Figure 1-20. No-assistant technique. (A) The trailing haptic is moved inferiorly up to the 6 o'clock position so that the vector forces come into play and the leading haptic now does not slip back into the eye. Surgeon leaves the leading haptic, and a glued IOL forceps introduced from the sideport incision grasps the trailing haptic. (B) The tip of trailing haptic is transferred to the second forceps using the handshake technique. (C) Tip of the trailing haptic is caught with the glued IOL forceps. (D) Trailing haptic is externalized. Finally, both haptics are externalized without the help of an assistant. (Reprinted with permission from Dr. Agarwal's Eye Hospital.)

inferiorly up to the 6 o'clock position, which ensures that no external forces are acting on the leading haptic that could cause it to slip inside. The surgeon leaves the leading haptic and then introduces the glued IOL forceps from the sideport incision. The tip of the trailing haptic is then transferred to the second forceps (Figure 1-20). Then, the surgeon enters the eye from the other sclerotomy site with the glued IOL forceps and catches the tip of the trailing haptic using the handshake technique. The trailing haptic is then pulled out and externalized.

WORKING WITHOUT AN ASSISTANT

The glued IOL technique requires an assistant to hold the haptics of the IOL once they have been externalized through the sclerotomies.[14] If an assistant is not available, it is likely that the externalized haptic will be

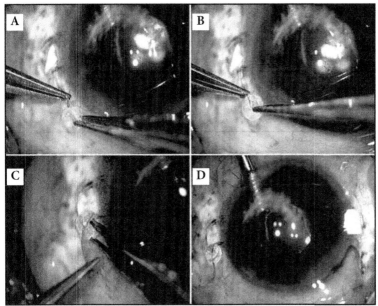

Figure 1-21. Beiko's/Steinert's modification. (A, B) Haptic passed through the narrow opening in the silicone tire of an iris hook. (C) Haptic passed fully. (D) Silicone tire of iris hook prevents the haptic from slipping back into the vitreous cavity. (Reprinted with permission from Dr. Agarwal's Eye Hospital.)

pulled into the eye once the second haptic is externalized. To prevent the migration of the first haptic into the eye, Dr. George Beiko recommended using a silicone tire (Figure 1-21). This silicone tire is readily available from a Mackool capsular support system (Impex Surgical) or MST capsular support (Microsurgical Technology, Inc). Placing the silicone tire on the haptic provides support for the haptic while other procedures are performed. Dr. Steven Safran performed the same technique using a small bit of the intravenous tubing.

OHTA'S Y-FIXATION TECHNIQUE

Dr. Toshihiko Ohta created a simplified, safer method of sutureless, intrascleral PC IOL fixation called the Y-fixation technique. With this technique, a Y-shaped incision is made in the sclera, and a 23-gauge MVR knife is used to create the sclerotomy instead of a needle. The Y-shaped incision eliminates the need to raise a lamellar scleral flap. The idea here is to create 2 Y-shaped incisions 2 mm from the limbus exactly 180 degrees apart diagonally. A scleral tunnel is made parallel to the limbus at the end of the Y-shaped incision, which helps improve wound closure.

HAPTIC RE-EXTERNALIZATION IN CASES OF INADEQUATELY EXTERNALIZED HAPTIC

While all these maneuvers are being done, some vitreous might be in the sclerotomy site. Vitrectomy should be done around the sclerotomy and then the IOL position should be assessed. The lens must be stable without anyone holding the IOL. If the haptic is slipping back, either of the following is possible:

- The eye is large and has a large WTW diameter, in which case a vertical glued IOL must be done.

- The sclerotomy is too far back so very little haptic has been externalized.

If the haptics are slipping back, a fresh sclerotomy[30,31] should be made more anterior to the previous one and the haptic pushed back into the vitreous cavity. Using the handshake technique, the haptic should be grasped and re-externalized through the fresh anterior sclerotomy. Once again, an assessment should be made as to whether the IOL is stable without tucking and gluing.

A key factor in the stability of glued intrascleral haptic fixation of PC IOLs is the length of the haptic tuck into the intrascleral tunnel. We need about 2 to 3 mm of haptic externalized so that enough haptic is tucked and postoperative dislocation does not occur. A sclerotomy that is unintentionally displaced posteriorly can move the plane of the entire PC IOL posteriorly. As a result, a shorter length of haptic is available to be tucked into the tunnel, which can lead to instability of the IOL, especially in larger eyes in which there is already less haptic to tuck. In addition, if only one side of the sclerotomy is displaced posteriorly, it can lead to a tilt of the IOL. If significant enough, it can cause visual symptoms. Therefore, placing both sclerotomies symmetrically at the appropriate distance from the limbus is important. In cases in which the sclerotomies are not symmetrical, we use a closed-chamber technique to externalize the haptic through a fresh sclerotomy (Figure 1-22).

A new sclerotomy is created anterior to the original sclerotomy, while being careful to leave an adequate bridge of tissue between the 2 sclerotomies to prevent them from uniting into a single large opening. After the sclerotomy is made, microforceps are passed through the sideport into the eye, and the haptic is again internalized in the eye. The tip of the tucked haptic is then grasped with the second microforceps using the handshake technique and brought out through the anteriorly placed sclerotomy.

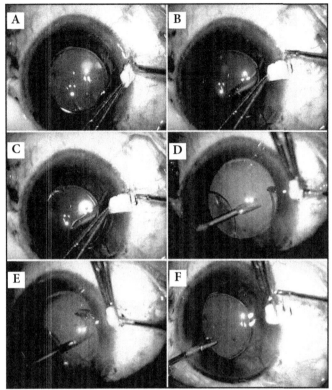

Figure 1-22. Haptic re-externalization. (A) Insufficient haptic externalized through a posteriorly displaced sclerotomy. A new sclerotomy is made anterior to the existing sclerotomy. (B) The haptic is grasped with microforceps. (C) The haptic is internalized into the vitreous cavity. (D) A second pair of microforceps are passed through the sideport for the handshake maneuver. (E) The first microforceps are passed through the new anterior sclerotomy, and the internalized haptic is grasped at the very tip using the handshake technique. (F) The haptic is re-externalized through the anterior sclerotomy. (Reprinted with permission from Dr. Agarwal's Eye Hospital.)

SCHARIOTH SCLERAL POCKET AND INTRASCLERAL HAPTIC TUCK

Dr. Gabor Scharioth created the first intrascleral haptic fixation in 2006. It is the intrascleral haptic fixation that gives stability to the IOL. A 26-gauge needle is bent so that it is like a keratome (Figure 1-23). The 26-gauge needle then creates a scleral tunnel at the edge of the flap where the haptic is externalized (Figure 1-24). The haptic is then flexed and tucked into the scleral pocket.

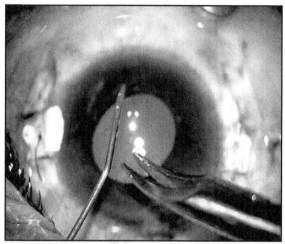

Figure 1-23. Twenty-six–gauge needle bent like a keratome. (Reprinted with permission from Dr. Agarwal's Eye Hospital.)

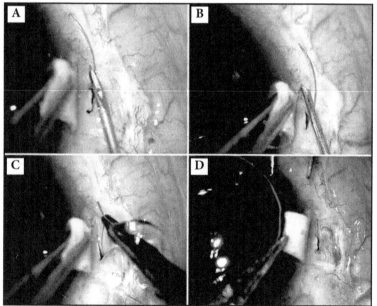

Figure 1-24. Scharioth scleral pocket creation with intrascleral haptic tuck. (A) A 26-gauge needle creating a scleral tunnel at the edge of the flap where the haptic is externalized. (B) Scharioth scleral pocket. (C) Haptic flexed to be tucked into the scleral pocket. (D) Haptic tucked in the scleral pocket. (Reprinted with permission from Dr. Agarwal's Eye Hospital.)

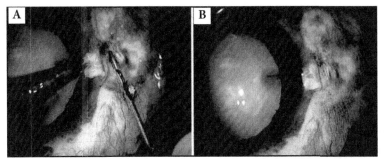

Figure 1-25. Marked Scharioth scleral pocket created before IOL implantation. (A) A 26-gauge needle is marked with the marker pen to leave a mark in the sclera where the scleral pocket is created; this can be done before opening the eye as it will have to be done adjacent to the area where the sclerotomy will be made. (B) Marked scleral pocket created. It is now easy to see where the scleral pocket is located. Another option is to pass a rod in the area of the sclera pocket to check its location. (Reprinted with permission from Dr. Agarwal's Eye Hospital.)

Alternatively, the Scharioth scleral pocket can be marked and created even before the eye is opened. The 26-gauge needle is marked with the marker pen (Figure 1-25) to leave a mark in the sclera where the scleral pocket is created. This can be done adjacent to the area where the sclerotomy will be made. It is now easy to see where the scleral pocket is located. Another option is to pass a rod in the area of the scleral pocket to check its location.

AIR IN THE ANTERIOR CHAMBER

Air is now injected into the AC, and the fluid from the infusion cannula is turned off (Figure 1-26). The fibrin glue has to work in a dry area so the fluid has to be turned off; otherwise, fluid might keep coming from the sclerotomy site. Once fluid is turned off, intraoperative hypotony and also postoperative hypotony are possible. To prevent this, we inject air in the AC to have a firm globe intra- and postoperatively. At the end of the case, when the speculum is removed, one should check for any hypotony and, if present, inject some fluid through the clear corneal incision to distend the eyeball.

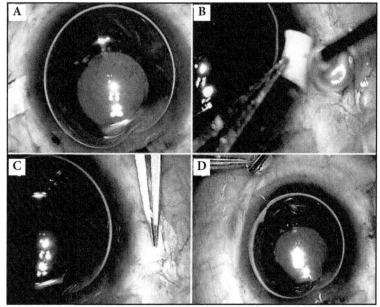

Figure 1-26. Fibrin glue application. (A) Air in AC. (B) Fibrin glue applied under the flaps. (C) Scleral flaps stuck. (D) Fibrin glue applied to seal the conjunctiva. (Reprinted with permission from Dr. Agarwal's Eye Hospital.)

ROLE OF FIBRIN GLUE

The fibrin glue plays a multifactorial role in glued IOL surgery:

- It helps seal the haptic to the sclera, which gives extra support to the intrascleral haptic tuck. One should remember that the key is the intrascleral pocket tuck of the haptic and not the glue.

- It seals the flaps so that there is no opening from inside the eye to the outside. This prevents any chance of endophthalmitis even some years later.

- It prevents any trabeculectomy opening because the flaps are secured firmly.

- It helps seal the cut conjunctiva.

- It helps seal the clear corneal incisions.

POSTOPERATIVE REGIMEN

Patients must be followed postoperatively because these are worst-case scenarios (Figure 1-27). They need postoperative antibiotic steroids for

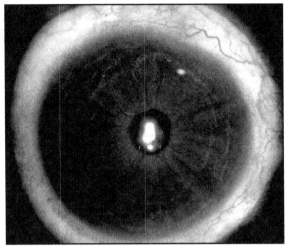

Figure 1-27. Glued IOL done in right eye (1.5 years postoperative). (Reprinted with permission from Dr. Agarwal's Eye Hospital.)

6 weeks. If there is temporary elevation of intraocular pressure, anti-glaucoma medications can be given. If the patient has a reaction, subconjunctival antibiotic-steroids may also be given. If there is hypotony, one can put the patient on systemic steroids.

STABILITY OF THE IOL HAPTIC

Because the flaps are manually created, the rough opposing surfaces of the flap and bed heal rapidly and firmly around the haptic, helped by the fibrin glue early on. The major uncertainty here is the stability of the fibrin matrix in vivo. Numerous animal studies have revealed that the fibrin glue is still present 4 to 6 weeks after surgery. Because postoperative fibrosis starts early, the flaps become stuck secondary to fibrosis even before full degradation of the glue. The ensuing fibrosis acts to make a firm scaffold around the haptic, which also prevents movement along the long axis (Figure 1-28A). To further stabilize the IOL, we tuck the haptic tip into the scleral wall through a tunnel, which prevents all movement of the haptic along the transverse axis as well (Figure 1-28B). The stability of the lens first comes through the tucking of the haptics in the scleral pocket created. The tissue glue then gives it extra stability and also seals the flap down. Externalization of the greater part of the haptic along its curvature stabilizes the axial positioning of the IOL and thereby prevents any IOL tilt.

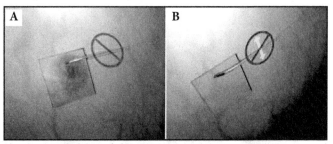

Figure 1-28. Stability of the IOL. (A) Long-axis movement is prevented by the tissue glue. (B) Transverse-axis movement is prevented by the scleral tuck. (Reprinted with permission from Dr. Agarwal's Eye Hospital.)

ADVANTAGES

This fibrin glue-assisted sutureless PC IOL implantation technique would be useful in myriad clinical situations, in which sclera-fixated IOLs are indicated, such as luxated IOL, dislocated IOL, zonulopathy, or secondary IOL implantation because of the following:

1. No special IOLs are required.

2. There is no tilt. Externalization of the greater part of the haptic along its curvature stabilizes the axial positioning of the IOL and thereby prevents any IOL tilt.

3. There is less pseudophacodonesis. When the eye moves, it acquires kinetic energy from its muscles and attachments, and the energy is dissipated to the internal fluids as it stops. Thus, pseudophacodonesis is the result of oscillations of the fluids in the anterior and posterior segments of the eye. These oscillations result in shearing forces on the corneal endothelium and vitreous motion, which lead to permanent damage. Because the IOL haptic is stuck beneath the flap, it would prevent the further movement of the haptic and thereby reduce pseudophacodonesis (Figure 1-29). Suture-fixated IOLs intend to simulate the crystalline lens–bag–zonule complex, which, because of its 360-degree attachment to the ciliary area, is a trampoline-like structure. However, the prolene sutures (2 or 4, depending on the technique) rather act as a hammock, which provides lesser torsional stability than the natural state. We feel that the difference from sutured secondary PC IOL lies in the rigid, nonelastic attachment of the IOL to the ciliary area with the glued IOL technique, which reduces the torsional and oscillatory freedom of the implant because the resultant IOL-haptic-ciliary body complex is more stable than the IOL–haptic–suture–ciliary body complex of

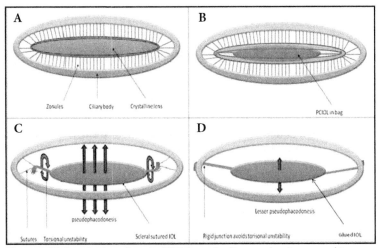

Figure 1-29. Pseudophacodonesis. (A) Schematic diagram showing normal trampoline line arrangement of ciliary body, zonules, and crystalline lens in a normal eye. (B) Schematic diagram showing the change in the case of a pseudophakic eye with an in-the-bag IOL. (C) A pseudophakic eye with a sutured sclera-fixated IOL: increased torsional instability and increased pseudophacodonesis due to ciliary body-suture-haptic attachment. (D) A pseudophakic eye with a glued IOL: reduced torsional instability and lesser pseudophacodonesis due to rigid ciliary body-haptic-optic attachment. (Reprinted with permission from Dr. Agarwal's Eye Hospital.)

the suture-fixated IOLs. This same biomechanical model is the reason for lesser pseudophacodonesis seen after glued IOL in comparison to suture-fixated IOLs.

4. Uveitis-glaucoma-hyphema (UGH) syndrome occurs less often. We expect less incidence of UGH syndrome in fibrin glue-assisted IOL implantation compared with sutured sclera-fixated IOL. In the former, the IOL is well stabilized and stuck onto the scleral bed, and thereby has decreased intraocular mobility, whereas in the latter, there is increased possibility of IOL movement or persistent rub over the ciliary body.

5. No suture-related complications. Visually significant complications due to late subluxation, which has been known to occur in sutured sclera-fixated IOL, may also be prevented because sutures are completely avoided in this technique. Another important advantage of this technique is the prevention of suture-related complications, such as suture erosion, suture knot exposure, or dislocation of IOL, after suture disintegration or a broken suture.

6. Speed and ease of surgery.

CAMERA ANALOGY AND SLOW MOTION VIDEOS

To understand why the glued IOL works better than the sutured-IOL or AC-IOL procedure, let us think of a camera. If we break the lens of the camera, fix it back to the camera body with sutures, and take photos, the picture quality will not be good because the lens would be moving. This is what happens in an eye with a sutured IOL because there is pseudophacodonesis. If we glued the lens to the camera body, both the lens and the body of the camera would move in unison. This is what happens after glued IOL surgery; there is no pseudophacodonesis, which provides better picture quality. The same can be shown through a slow-motion camera application.

Subtle intraocular movements such as iridodonesis, phacodonesis, and pseudophacodonesis are often unappreciated or unnoticed.[25] The newest iPhone (Apple) models support the recording of high-speed photography that allows capturing slow-motion video with the native camera application (app). This nifty feature was first introduced as a major part of the iPhone 5s camera and is able to shoot 720p (progressive scan; noninterlaced) movies at 120 frames per second (fps). This feature was enhanced in the iPhone 6, and the slow-motion recording imparts 240 fps. Human eyes are accustomed to videos that are played at 24 to 30 fps. Slow motion captures a bunch of pictures very quickly, and adjusting the smartphone camera to 120 fps (iPhone 5s) or 240 fps (iPhone 6) sets the recording of at least 120 or 240 images per second, respectively. When this video runs, it typically plays back at an eyeball-friendly 24 to 30 fps. In other words, 120 images are played at the speed at which the human eye is receptive. The huge excess of 120 images that were filmed in 1 second of real shooting lasts for 4 seconds or more ($30 \times 4 = 120$) on the screen. Thus, slow motion is derived. Detection of pseudophacodonesis is another important aspect of "slo-mo" recording. It has a clinical implication of explaining the process of subsequent vitreous disturbance and cystoid macular edema (CME). Demonstration of the slow displacing movement of the IOL in the eye with ocular movement in cases of an AC IOL and iris claw IOL may lead to rubbing of the IOL on the iris surface or a hammock-like movement. Potential movement of the IOL may cause disturbance in the vitreous cavity, or in cases of AC IOL, it may cause a release of inflammatory tissue from the iris leading to prolonged CME. An improperly fitted AC IOL with marked pseudophacodonesis should be explanted and an appropriately sized AC IOL should be placed inside the eye. High-fps recording of glued IOL does not demonstrate pseudophacodonesis. This may be because of the intrascleral tucking of the haptics, which prevents any movement of the IOL. Postoperative detection of pseudophacodonesis in glued IOL may be present in cases with improper tucking. In such a scenario, the scleral flaps from glued IOL surgery should be lifted and proper tucking should be done.

REFERENCES

1. Maggi R, Maggi C. Sutureless scleral fixation of intraocular lenses. *J Cataract Refract Surg.* 1997;23(9):1289-1294.
2. Gabor SG, Pavilidis MM. Sutureless intrascleral posterior chamber intraocular lens fixation. *J Cataract Refract Surg.* 2007;33(11):1851-1854.
3. Agarwal A, Kumar DA, Jacob S, Baid C, Agarwal A, Srinivasan S. Fibrin glue–assisted sutureless posterior chamber intraocular lens implantation in eyes with deficient posterior capsules. *J Cataract Refract Surg.* 2008;34(9):1433-1438.
4. Kumar DA, Agarwal A, Prakash G, Jacob S, Saravanan Y, Agarwal A. Glued posterior chamber IOL in eyes with deficient capsular support: a retrospective analysis of 1-year post-operative outcomes. *Eye (Lond).* 2010;24(7):1143-1148.
5. Prakash G, Kumar DA, Jacob S, Kumar KS, Agarwal A, Agarwal A. Anterior segment optical coherence tomography–aided diagnosis and primary posterior chamber intraocular lens implantation with fibrin glue in traumatic phacocele with scleral perforation. *J Cataract Refract Surg.* 2009;35(4):782-784.
6. Prakash G, Jacob S, Kumar DA, Narsimhan S, Agarwal A, Agarwal A. Femtosecond assisted keratoplasty with fibrin glue–assisted sutureless posterior chamber lens implantation: a new triple procedure. *J Cataract Refract Surg.* 2009;35(6):973-979.
7. Nair V, Kumar DA, Prakash G, Jacob S, Agarwal A, Agarwal A. Bilateral spontaneous in-the-bag anterior subluxation of PC IOL managed with glued IOL technique: a case report. *Eye Contact Lens.* 2009;35(4):215-217.
8. Agarwal A, Kumar DA, Prakash G, et al. Fibrin glue–assisted sutureless posterior chamber intraocular lens implantation in eyes with deficient posterior capsules [reply to letter]. *J Cataract Refract Surg.* 2009;35(5):795-796.
9. Kumar DA, Agarwal A, Jacob S, Prakash G, Agarwal A, Sivagnanam S. Repositioning of the dislocated intraocular lens with sutureless 20-gauge vitrectomy. *Retina.* 2010;30(4):682-687.
10. Kumar DA, Agarwal A, Prakash G, Jacob S. Managing total aniridia with aphakia using a glued iris prosthesis. *J Cataract Refract Surg.* 2010;36(5):864-865.
11. Kumar DA, Agarwal A, Gabor SG, et al. Sutureless sclera fixated posterior chamber intraocular lens [letter to editor]. *J Cataract Refract Surg.* 2011;37(11):2089-2090.
12. Agarwal A, Jacob S, Kumar DA, et al. Handshake technique for glued intrascleral haptic fixation of a posterior chamber intraocular lens. *J Cataract Refract Surg.* 2013;39(3):317-322.
13. Narang P, Narang S. Glue-assisted intrascleral fixation of posterior chamber intraocular lens. *Indian J Ophthalmol.* 2013;61(4):163-167.
14. Beiko G, Steinert R. Modification of externalized haptic support of glued intraocular lens technique. *J Cataract Refract Surg.* 2013;39(3):323-325.
15. Sinha R, Bali SJ, Sharma N, Titiyal JS. Fibrin glue-assisted fixation of decentered posterior chamber intraocular lens. *Eye Contact Lens.* 2012; 38(1):68-71.
16. McKee Y, Price FW Jr, Feng MT, et al. Implementation of the posterior chamber intraocular lens intrascleral haptic fixation technique (glued intraocular lens) in a United States practice: outcomes and insights. *J Cataract Refract Surg.* 2014;40(12):2099-2105.

17. Narang P. Modified method of haptic externalization of posterior chamber intraocular lens in fibrin glue-assisted intrascleral fixation: no-assistant technique. *J Cataract Refract Surg.* 2013;39(1):4-7.

18. Ganekal S, Venkataratnam S, Dorairaj S, Jhanji V. Comparative evaluation of suture-assisted and fibrin glue-assisted scleral fixated intraocular lens implantation. *J Refract Surg.* 2012; 28(4):249-252.

19. Scharioth GB, Prasad S, Georgalas I, et al. Intermediate results of sutureless intrascleral posterior chamber intraocular lens fixation. *J Cataract Refract Surg.* 2010;36(2):254-259.

20. Kumar DA, Agarwal A, Prakash G, et al. Evaluation of intraocular lens tilt with anterior segment optical coherence tomography. *Am J Ophthalmol.* 2011;151(3):406-412.

21. Kumar DA, Agarwal A, Packiyalakshmi S, et al. Complications and visual outcomes after glued foldable intraocular lens implantation in eyes with inadequate capsules. *J Cataract Refract Surg.* 2013;39(8):1211-1218.

22. Kumar DA, Agarwal A, Jacob S, Agarwal A. Glued transscleral intraocular lens exchange for anterior chamber lenses in complicated eyes: analysis of indications and results. *Am J Ophthalmol.* 2013;156(6):1125-1133.

23. Ashok Kumar D, Agarwal A, Agarwal A, Chandrasekar R. Clinical outcomes of glued transscleral fixated intraocular lens in functionally one-eyed patients. *Eye Contact Lens.* 2014;40(4):e23-e28.

24. Kumar DA, Agarwal A, Agarwal A, Chandrasekar R, Priyanka V. Long-term assessment of tilt of glued intraocular lenses: an optical coherence tomography analysis 5 years after surgery. *Ophthalmology.* 2015;122(1):48-55.

25. Narang P, Agarwal A, Sanu AS. Technique to detect subtle intraocular movements: enhanced frames per second recording (slow motion) using smartphones. *J Cataract Refract Surg.* 2015;41(6):1321-1323.

26. Ladi, JS, Shah NA. Vertical fixation with fibrin glue-assisted secondary posterior chamber intraocular lens implantation in a case of surgical aphakia. *Indian J Ophthalmol.* 2013;61(3):126-129.

27. Jackson MR, MacPhee MJ, Drohan WN, Alving BM. Fibrin sealant: current and potential clinical applications. *Blood Coagul Fibrinolysis.* 1996;7(8):737-746.

28. Matras H. Fibrin seal: the state of the art. *J Oral Maxillofac Surg.* 1985; 43(8):605-611.

29. Agarwal A, Agarwal A, Jacob S, Narang P. Comprehending IOL signs and the significance in glued IOL surgery. *J Refract Surg.* 2013;29(2):79.

30. Kumar DA, Agarwal A. Glued intraocular lens: a major review on surgical technique and results. *Curr Opin Ophthalmol.* 2013;24(1):21-29.

31. Jacob S, Agarwal A, Agarwal A, Narasimhan S. Closed-chamber haptic reexternalization for posteriorly displaced sclerotomy and inadequate haptic tuck in glued posterior chamber intraocular lenses. *J Cataract Refract Surg.* 2015;41(2):268-271.

2

Glued IOL Surgery for Subluxated IOLs and Other Challenging Cases

Ashvin Agarwal, MS and
Amar Agarwal, MS, FRCS, FRCOphth

Dislocation of an intraocular lens (IOL) into the vitreous can occur as an early or late complication arising from posterior capsular rupture during phacoemulsification.[1] Management of such a situation with available instruments without compromising the visual outcome remains a challenge. Traditionally, dislocated IOLs have been managed by repositioning either the same or a different IOL with sutured scleral fixation or replacing the lens with an anterior chamber (AC) IOL (Figures 2-1 through 2-4). Such a procedure is routinely combined with conventional pars plana vitrectomy.

We use the glued IOL technique for subluxated IOLs.[2-13] We can reposition the dislocated IOL in the posterior chamber (PC) with transscleral fixation of haptics, intralamellar scleral tuck, and fibrin glue-assisted flap closure. If the IOL is an AC IOL or a single-piece foldable IOL, then the IOL is explanted, and a new 3-piece PC IOL is glued in place. The glued IOL procedure can be performed in various worst-case scenarios to help the patient achieve satisfactory vision.[14-19]

Agarwal A, ed.
A Video Textbook of Glued IOLs (pp 37-60).
© 2016 Taylor & Francis Group.

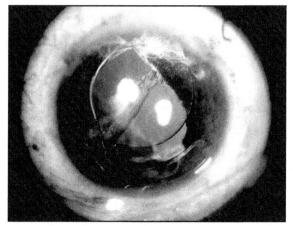

Figure 2-1. AC IOL.

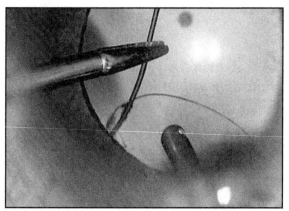

Figure 2-2. Dislocated 3-piece sutured IOL. The same IOL is glued back in place using the handshake technique.

This chapter provides various advanced techniques. Depending on accessibility to instruments and surgeon comfort, a retinal surgeon may be managing subluxated crystalline or dislocated IOLs.

SUBLUXATED 3-PIECE IOL

The haptics of a subluxated 3-piece IOL are very easy to externalize through the sclerotomies without explanting the IOL (Figures 2-5 and 2-6).

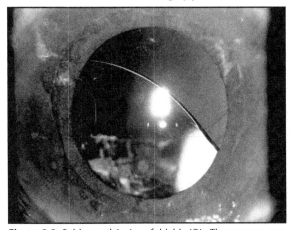

Figure 2-3. Subluxated 1-piece foldable IOL. The surgeon can make a scleral tunnel to explant the IOL and glue in a fresh 3-piece PC IOL.

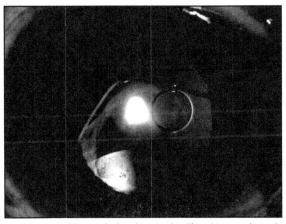

Figure 2-4. Subluxated plate haptic IOL. This IOL is explanted, and a 3-piece IOL is glued in place. These lenses are not sutured because sutures create pseudophacodonesis.

The reason is that the haptics are quite malleable and so can be externalized easily. The haptic must be held with the glued IOL forceps while vitrectomy is being done with the other hand so that there is no vitreous traction. Remember to grab the tip of the haptic while externalizing so that the haptic is not deformed. The handshake technique helps to achieve this goal. Once the haptics are externalized, they can be tucked into the Scharioth pockets and glued.

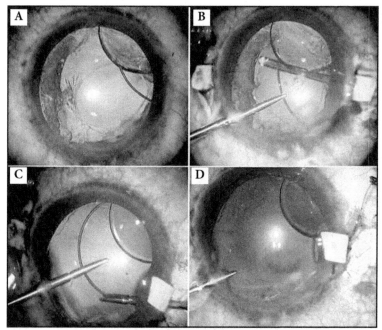

Figure 2-5. Subluxated 3-piece IOL glued into place (part 1). (A) A 3-piece IOL above the rhexis is still subluxated. (B) Scleral flaps are made 180 degrees apart. One hand holds the haptic with the glued IOL forceps while the other is performing vitrectomy. The capsule remnants are removed because they are not needed for the glued IOL. (C) The handshake technique is used to catch the tip of the haptic. Notice the trocar cannula on the upper right. Fluid is needed in the eye at all times. A trocar AC maintainer may also be used. (D) One haptic is externalized.

ONE-PIECE NONFOLDABLE POLYMETHYLMETHACRYLATE SUBLUXATED IOL

It is a bit tricky to reposition a single-piece, nonfoldable polymethylmethacrylate (PMMA) IOL using the glued IOL technique because haptics can break during the surgery (Figure 2-7). The scleral flaps should be created and infusion fixed before the vitrectomy is performed. Using 2 glued IOL forceps and the handshake technique, each haptic is externalized through the sclerotomies under the scleral flaps. They are then tucked and glued in the Scharioth tunnels. If the haptic breaks during removal, it can be explanted through a scleral tunnel incision, and a fresh 3-piece PC IOL may be glued in.

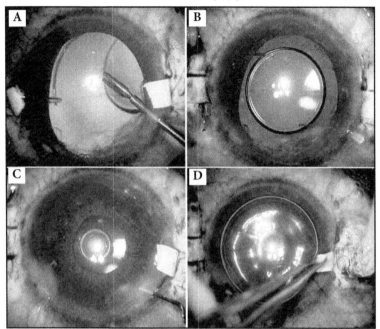

Figure 2-6. Subluxated 3-piece IOL glued into place (part 2). (A) The second haptic is caught with the handshake technique. (B) Both haptics are externalized. (C) Both haptics are tucked in Scharioth pocket. (D) Air in the AC, fluid is switched off, and glue applied. The air prevents any hypotony.

SUBLUXATED CAPSULAR BAG—IOL COMPLEX

Subluxated capsular bag–IOL complex cases are tricky to handle (Figure 2-8). In such cases, there may be thick Soemmering's rings. A Sommering's ring should be managed by using the glued IOL scaffold technique. Vitrectomy can be done, but sometimes the rings are quite thick and can fall down into the vitreous cavity. It might be better to explant the complex through a scleral tunnel incision. Once it is explanted and vitrectomy is done, a 3-piece IOL can be glued into place.

ONE-PIECE FOLDABLE IOL

A single-piece foldable IOL cannot be fixed and glued because a firm haptic to tuck and glue into the sclera is required for the glued IOL technique.

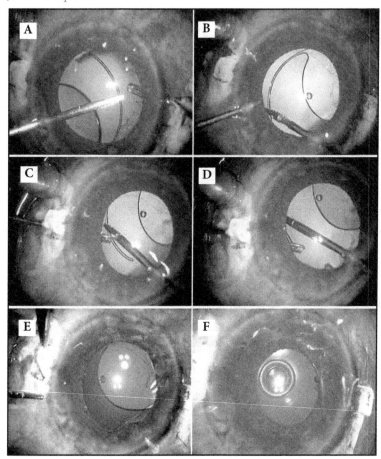

Figures 2-7. Management of a subluxated one-piece PMMA nonfoldable IOL. (A) Subluxated single-piece PMMA IOL. Vitrectomy is performed. Note that one haptic is held with the glued IOL forceps to prevent the IOL from falling down while the vitrectomy is done. (B) One haptic caught with the glued IOL forceps. (C) Second forceps passed through the sclerotomy under the scleral flap to grab the haptic using the handshake technique. (D) Haptic tip grasped to externalize the haptic. (E) Haptic externalized. One should be careful when doing this in a single-piece nonfoldable PMMA IOL as the haptic can break. (F) Both haptics externalized and tucked. Glue will then be applied. Note the well-centered IOL.

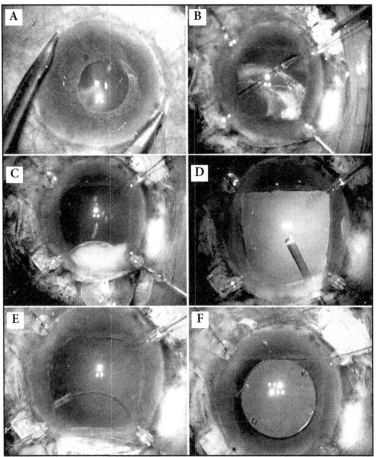

Figure 2-8. Management of a subluxated capsular bag–IOL complex. (A) Subluxated capsular bag–IOL complex. Measure the white-to-white diameter of the cornea and, if the horizontal is more than 11 mm, perform a vertical glued IOL. (B) Scleral flaps made, infusion fixed, and vitrectomy done. One hand holds the haptic with glued IOL forceps to prevent the bag–IOL complex from falling down. (C) Explantation of the bag–IOL complex through a scleral tunnel incision. The surgeon can perform a vitrectomy and chew up the bag, but, in some cases, there are thick Soemmering's rings that are difficult to chew and can fall down onto the retina. In such cases, it might be more prudent to explant the entire complex. (D) Vitrectomy. (E) Glued IOL technique started with a 3-piece IOL. (F) Haptics externalized and tucked. Glue is applied.

The haptics in a single-piece foldable IOL are too flexible to tuck and glue. In such cases, the IOL should be explanted and a 3-piece IOL refixated with the glued IOL technique. We do not suture these IOLs because the results of the glued IOL procedure are much better. Although there is a slightly larger incision for explanting the IOL, we still prefer it to suturing an existing foldable single-piece IOL.

EXTRUSION CANNULA ASSISTED LEVITATION FOR A DROPPED IOL

IOLs that are dislocated into the PC have always been a cause of concern and are a known complication following a PC rupture. Improper sulcus fixation, dislocation/subluxation of the bag–complex, or improper judgement of the integrity of the PC intraoperatively can lead to this complicated scenario. Dislocation of the IOL not only makes the patient aphakic, but also can cause complications related to the dropped IOL. Therefore, it is mandatory to explant or reposition the IOL, which in itself has its own complications and requires a major vitreoretinal intervention.

PERFLUOROCARBON LIQUIDS

Dr. Stanley Chang popularized the use of perfluorocarbon liquids (PFCLs) for the surgical treatment of various vitreoretinal disorders. Due to their heavier-than-water properties and their ease of intraocular injection and removal, PFCLs are highly effective for flattening detached retina, tamponading a retinal tear, limiting intraocular hemorrhage, and floating dropped crystalline lens fragments and a dislocated IOL. We generally do not use PFCL for dislocated IOLs, but if it is used, the PFCL must be removed at the end of surgery.

CHANDELIER ILLUMINATION

Visualization of the fundus during vitrectomy is achieved by using chandelier illumination, in which xenon light is fixed to a trocar cannula (Figure 2-9). This light provides excellent illumination and enables the surgeon to perform a proper bimanual vitrectomy because a handheld endoilluminator is not necessary. An inverter must be used if a widefield lens is used. The

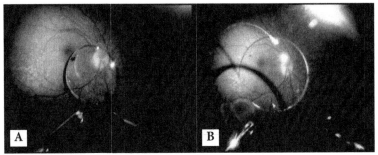

Figure 2-9. (A) An intraoperactive picture, showing the chandelier technique being performed in a completely dislocated IOL in the vitreous. (B) Internal illumination is from the halogen light source attached to the infusion cannula (chandelier illumination).

SuperMacula lens (Volk Optical) provides better stereopsis so that there is no difficulty in holding the IOL with diamond-tipped forceps. A noncontact viewing system such as a BIOM (Oculus Surgical) may also be used.

When using the chandelier illumination system, the surgeon can hold the IOL with the forceps in one hand and with the other hold a vitrectomy probe to cut the adhesions of the vitreous, thus performing a bimanual vitrectomy. The handshake technique can be performed by using 2 forceps to hold the lens.

EXTRUSION CANNULA

The extrusion cannula has been used extensively for drainage of subretinal fluid by posterior segment surgeons. The flexible sleeve of the extrusion cannula helps to reach the subretinal space effectively. In our practice, we use extrusion cannulas without sleeves for levitating dropped IOLs.[14] Removal of the sleeve provides a wider area for adherence and subsequent creation of effective suction to the IOL.

SURGICAL TECHNIQUE

After a standard 3-port pars plana vitrectomy procedure (Figure 2-10) and clearance of all the vitreolenticular adhesions, the sleeveless extrusion cannula is connected to the vacuum of the vitreotome. The extrusion cannula is introduced and brought close to the anterior surface of the optic of the IOL (Figure 2-11). Effective suction is generated by pressing the foot

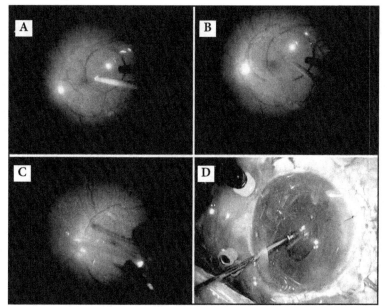

Figure 2-10. Extrusion cannula for dislocated IOL. (A) Vitrectomy performed for a dropped IOL. (B) A sleeveless extrusion cannula is placed over the optic of the IOL to lift it by suction. (C) The IOL is lifted by suction. (D) The IOL is brought anteriorly and the haptic is held with end-opening forceps.

pedal with a setting at around 300 mm Hg. The IOL is levitated and brought in to the midpupillary plane, where it is grasped by end-opening forceps introduced through the sideport incision. The IOL haptic must be grabbed in the anterior vitreous so that the IOL does not fall down (Figure 2-12). The IOL is then explanted or repositioned, depending on the integrity of the sulcus support and also on the type of IOL that is levitated. Glued intrascleral haptic fixation is our method of choice in patients who require explantation and a subsequent IOL implantation (Figure 2-13). Once externalized, the tips of the haptics are tucked through a Scharioth intralamellar scleral tunnel made with a 26-gauge needle at the point of externalization. The scleral flaps are then closed with fibrin glue.

ADVANTAGES OF THE GLUED IOL TECHNIQUE

Vitrectomy and IOL fixation through the pars plicata have been reported in special situations. Although there is a possible risk of intraoperative hyphema because the sclerotomy is through the pars plicata, it is rare.

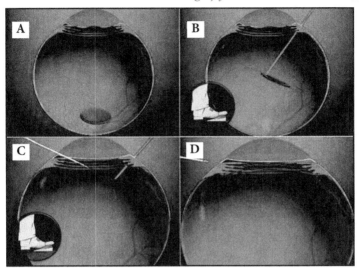

Figure 2-11. Illustration showing extrusion cannula assisted levitation. (A) PC IOL on the retina. (B) Extrusion cannula lifting the PC IOL. Foot pedal is pressed for suction. (C) Extrusion cannula brings the PC IOL under the iris. Foot pedal is pressed for suction. Glued IOL forceps grab the haptic so that the IOL does not fall. (D) PC IOL placed in sulcus if rhexis support is there or glued in place.

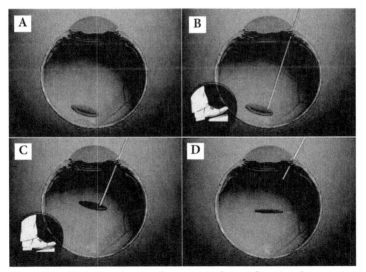

Figure 2-12. Illustration showing the wrong technique for using the extrusion cannula for lifting a dropped IOL. (A) PC IOL on the retina. (B) Extrusion cannula lifting the PC IOL. Foot pedal is pressed for suction. (C) Extrusion cannula brings the PC IOL under the iris. Foot pedal is pressed for suction. (D) IOL falls down because glued IOL forceps are not used to grab the haptic.

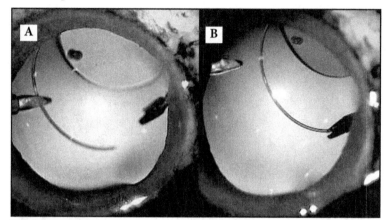

Figure 2-13. (A, B) Handshake technique. Intravitreal forceps are used to hold the haptic while the IOL is brought to the pupillary plane.

A sclerotomy wound can cause prolapsed and incarceration of uveal tissue and retinal fragments leading to vitreous traction and iatrogenic retinal breaks; however, in our experience, the postoperative ultrasound biomicroscopy showed no vitreous traction or retinal incarceration in the pars plicata ports. We have performed intralamellar tucking of the IOL haptic followed by fibrin glue application after externalization. We prefer glued IOL repositioning because the suture-related complications of scleral fixation IOL are reduced by this procedure. Because the IOL haptic is tucked in the scleral tunnel, it prevents further movement of the haptic, reducing pseudophacodonesis and minimizing slippage and late redislocation. Although complete scleral wound healing with collagen fibrils may take up to 3 months, the IOL remains very stable from the early postoperative period because the haptic is snugly placed inside an intralamellar scleral tunnel. The risk of retinal photic injury that is known to occur in sutured scleral fixation IOLs also is reduced with this technique because of the short surgical time. This new method avoids additional corneal incisions or multiple sclerotomies, and reduces surgical time and intraocular pressure fluctuation by maintaining a closed system.

COMBINED SURGICAL MANAGEMENT OF CAPSULAR AND IRIS DEFICIENCY WITH GLUED IOL: A GLUED IRIS PROSTHESIS AND THE GLUED IOL TECHNIQUE WITH PUPILLOPLASTY

Traumatic aniridia with combined lens injuries leading to aphakia is one of the sequelae after severe blunt trauma. Congenital aniridia with badly subluxated cataract also is not uncommon. Such conditions with iris and lens abnormalities lead to both cosmetic and optical defects. An intact iris diaphragm is essential because it reduces the optical aberrations arising from the crystalline lens and thereby increases the depth of focus. Thus, total aniridia is known to cause incapacitating glare and photophobia. Moreover, associated aphakia induces additional refractive problems to the existing defect. Managing aniridia and aphakia together is always challenging for a cataract surgeon. Iris reconstructive implants have been implanted intracapsularly in some cases of aniridia with capsular bag.[20] In eyes with partial aniridia, iris enclavation has been tried. However, in eyes with total aniridia with aphakia, transscleral fixation was an option.[16] We manage total aniridia and aphakia with an aniridia IOL implanted with the glued IOL technique. We also manage partial iris defects and aphakia with glued IOL and pupilloplasty.

Glued Iris Prosthesis

Aniridia is an ocular condition characterized by total or partial absence of iris. It can be congenital or acquired (Figure 2-14). The glued iris prosthesis designed by Dr. Kenneth Rosenthal is a PMMA aniridia IOL implanted with the glued IOL technique (Figure 2-15). We used the OV lens Style ANI5 (Intra Ocular Care) aniridia implant. The overall diameter of the implant is approximately 12.75 mm. The optic has a central clear zone of approximately 5 mm (clear optic zone) with a peripheral opaque or pigmented annulus of approximately 9.5 mm. The haptics are also made of PMMA with acute angulations, and there is an eyelet on both haptics for prolene suture placement during transscleral fixation.

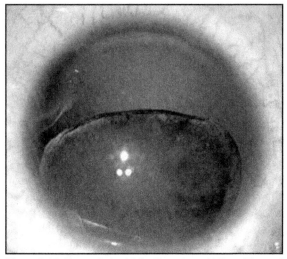

Figure 2-14. Congenital aniridia. Note the aniridia, subluxated colobomatous cataract, and stem cell deficiency. Patient also had glaucoma.

Surgical Technique for Glued Iris Prosthesis

Two partial-thickness scleral flaps approximately 2.5 × 2.5 mm are created exactly 180 degrees apart diagonally, approximately 1.0 mm from the limbus (see Figure 2-15). Infusion cannula or trocar AC maintainer is fixed. Superior 2.8-mm entry with the keratome is made and lensectomy is performed to remove the subluxated cataractous lens with a vitrectomy cutter. An anterior vitrectomy is completed to remove any vitreous traction. Two straight sclerotomies with an 18-gauge needle are made under the existing scleral flaps. The limbal incision is enlarged with a sharp keratome or corneoscleral scissors. The PMMA aniridia implant is then introduced through the limbal incision using McPherson forceps. End-gripping 25/23-gauge microrhexis forceps (Micro Surgical Technology) are passed through one of the sclerotomies to hold the tip of the haptic. The haptics are then externalized under the scleral flap. Precautions are taken during externalization because the angulation of the haptic with optic in the implant is different from the routine in-the-bag or sclera-fixated IOLs. A scleral tunnel is made with a 26-gauge needle at the point of externalization of the haptic and the haptic is tucked into the intralamellar scleral tunnel. The scleral flaps are then closed with Tisseel fibrin glue (Baxter). The infusion cannula or AC maintainer is then removed. The procedure also can be performed with 23-gauge trocar cannula infusion. The limbal wound is closed with

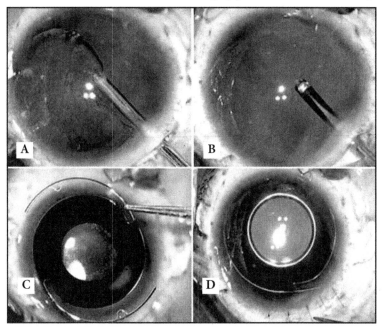

Figure 2-15. Aniridia glued IOL. (A) Congenital aniridia. Note the 2 scleral flaps and a third flap for trabeculectomy. The lensectomy has started. (B) Aniridia IOL implantation and the haptic tip caught with the glued IOL forceps. Note the trocar cannula in the upper-right corner for fluid infusion. (C) Aniridia IOL. (D) Both haptics tucked in Scharioth pockets. Fibrin glue is applied. The surgeon should be careful not to apply the fibrin glue in the trabeculectomy area. (Figures A and D are reprinted with permission from Kumar DA, Agarwal A, Prakash G, Jacob S. Managing total aniridia with aphakia using a glued iris prosthesis. *J Cataract Refract Surg.* 2010;36(5):864-865.)

10-0 monofilament nylon sutures. The conjunctiva is apposed with the fibrin glue. If there is glaucoma, a trabeculectomy or any antiglaucoma surgery can be done simultaneously. The same technique can be used in cases of acquired aniridia.

Glued IOL With Pupilloplasty

In cases of glued IOL with iridoplasty, the scleral flaps are created, followed by implantation of the 3-piece foldable IOL and intrascleral tuck of the haptics. The iridoplasty is then performed and the scleral flaps are closed with fibrin glue.

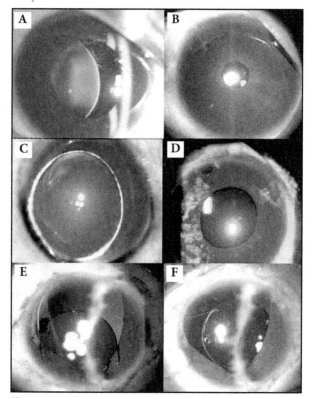

Figure 2-16. (A) IOL status in glued IOL follow-up in children. Preoperative picture of subluxated crystalline lens and (B) 2 years after surgery. (C) Preoperative clinical photograph of total subluxated lens with spherophakia and (D) 3 years after surgery. (E) Preoperative clinical photographs of decentered PC IOL and (F) 2 years after glued IOL surgery.

PEDIATRIC GLUED IOL

Pediatric eyes differ from those of adults due to their rapid growth and significant refractive changes in early childhood.[18] Therefore, IOL implantation after cataract surgery in these eyes should be matched to the growing and changing refraction. IOL implantation in eyes with large posterior capsular rent or ectopia lentis becomes further complicated due to lack of normal capsular support. Glued IOL works very well in pediatric eyes (Figure 2-16). In coloboma of the lens, even if the lens is clear, we perform lensectomy with glued IOL as these patients have aberropia and

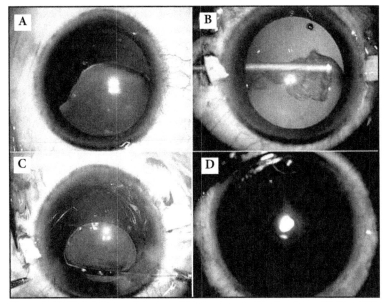

Figure 2-17. (A) Coloboma of the lens. (B) Lensectomy with vitrectomy. (C) Glued IOL implantation. (D) Postoperative picture.

once lensectomy is done the causative problem is solved and they see well (Figure 2-17).

One of the advantages of using the glued IOL technique in pediatric cases is that these IOLs are very sturdy and do not dislocate generally, so that is a long-term advantage for the child. In infants younger than 2 years, it is important to remember that the pars plana is very close to the limbus as the eye is developing, so always have the infusion all closer to the limbus (approximately 1 mm from the limbus). The same applies when one is operating on a microcornea eye.

Combined Silicone Oil Removal and Glued IOL Implantation in Eyes With Deficient Capsules

In eyes with previous vitreoretinal surgery requiring silicone oil injection, visual recovery is still a problem. Silicone oil injection has been widely used for long-term tamponade in complex surgeries, including those for

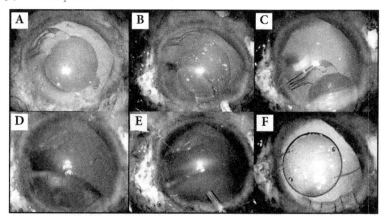

Figure 2-18. Silicone oil removal (SOR) with IOL explantation and glued IOL implantation. (A) Opacified IOL in an eye with silicone oil. (B) Two partial-thickness scleral flaps made and 23-gauge trocar cannula infusion fixed. (C) Corneolimbal incision made and the opacified IOL explanted. (D, E) SOR proceeded with the transpupillary method. (F) Glued IOL implantation done and extended limbal incision closed with sutures.

retinal detachment, proliferative vitreoretinopathy, vitreous hemorrhage, tractional retinal detachment, and traumatized eyes. However, silicone oil is associated with long-term complications, such as emulsification, glaucoma, keratopathy, and cataract formation. It is generally recommended to remove silicone oil 3 to 6 months after surgery, although there is still no definite guideline regarding the best time for silicone oil removal (SOR). The lens surgeries that are usually combined with SOR are the removal of a cataractous lens or the explantation of an opacified IOL.

SOR can be performed using a 23-gauge transconjunctival 3-port pars plana sclerotomy with motorized active suction with continuous infusion through the pars plana trocar. In cases where emulsified silicone oil is present, multiple air-fluid exchanges are performed, if possible, to ensure complete removal of the emulsified oil. In cases with silicone oil in the anterior chamber or inverse hypopyon, a thorough wash of the AC can be done with balanced salt solution after making a sideport incision. In eyes with an opacified IOL, the superior incision is extended and the IOL is explanted (Figure 2-18). If the eye is aphakic, one can remove the silicone oil when needed and implant a glued IOL at the same time (Figure 2-19).

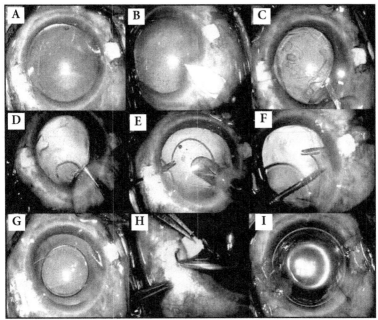

Figure 2-19. SOR with glued IOL implantation. (A) Two partial-thickness scleral flaps are made and 23-gauge trocar cannula inserted. (B) Corneolimbal incision made. (C) Transpupillary silicone oil removal done by gentle pressure on the posterior lip and keeping the infusion on. (D) Continuous passive SOR continued until the free fluid is visible. (E) Three-piece foldable IOL injected through the limbal wound, and the leading IOL haptic is captured by the glued IOL forceps via the sclerotomy. (F) Another haptic is externalized with the handshake technique. (G) Both the haptics externalized and the IOL centered. (H) IOL haptics tucked in intrascleral Scharioth tunnels. (I) Anterior chamber formed by air and scleral flaps apposed with fibrin glue.

MULTIFOCAL GLUED IOL

Multifocal IOL implantation for the correction of ametropia aims for good, unaided visual acuity for both near and distance.

ANGLE KAPPA

Angle kappa is the angle between the visual axis and the pupillary axis. It is clinically very important to the refractive surgeon because patients, especially hyperopic ones, have a large angle kappa and therefore the center of the pupil is no longer the point through which a fovea-centric ray of light passes. Thus, any treatment that is performed centered on the pupil results in a decentered ablation. This effect is more pronounced with corrections for astigmatism and higher-order aberrations if the surgeon does not compensate for angle kappa.

ANGLE KAPPA AND MULTIFOCAL IOLS

What role does angle kappa play for the cataract surgeon? We know that multifocal IOLs work by creating multiple focal points that focus for distance and near. We also know that patients with monofocal IOLs have traditionally been more satisfied with their visual outcome with regard to postoperative blurry vision, halos, glare, and decreased contrast sensitivity. Multifocal IOLs have been associated with these symptoms despite uneventful surgery with the IOL well centered in the bag. Many factors have been proposed for these phenomena, the most important of which is a decrease in the intensity of light falling on the retina due to splitting up of incident light into multiple focal points as well as superimposition of the defocused image onto the focused image. Although these factors are common to all patients, not all patients are affected equally by the symptoms. One of the factors proposed to account for this difference in symptoms is differing degrees of neuroadaptation. Other factors include IOL decentration, retained lens fragments, posterior capsular opacification, poor ocular surface, and postoperative residual refractive error. The newer-model multifocal IOLs have fewer symptoms associated with them.

Little research has focused on angle kappa as a factor. Angle kappa is the distance between the center of the pupil and the light reflex. The vertex normal or the light reflex is near the visual axis at the corneal plane. Angle kappa can be measured with the synoptophore or by using the Orbscan II (Bausch + Lomb). The average angle kappa is ±5 degrees. The effect of angle kappa on multifocal IOLs has been evaluated previously by attempting iridoplasty to make the pupil concentric to the center of the IOL, which could theoretically increase the effect of higher-order aberrations because of an increase in the pupil size. Angle kappa values may be considered in preoperative decision making in cases of multifocal IOL implantation. The reason for this association needs to be evaluated in detail with simulation methods, such as ray tracing, to confirm whether edge effect from the anterior IOL surface's rings may be responsible. A higher angle kappa indicates that the actual misalignment between the anatomical center of the pupil–IOL complex (through which a fovea-centric ray should pass, ideally) and the visual axis may be large enough to misalign the ray onto a ring edge (Figure 2-20).

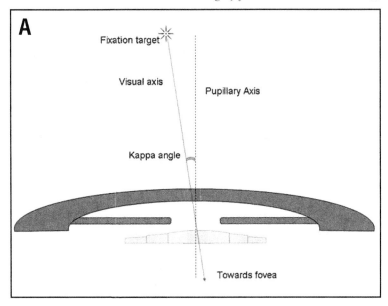

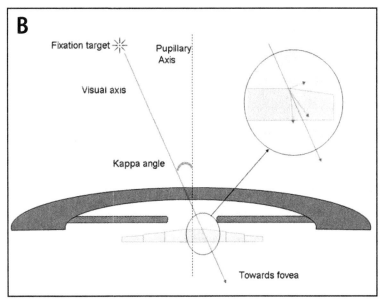

Figure 2-20. Angle kappa and multifocal IOL. (A) Schematic ray diagram showing the incident ray passing through the central area in an eye with small angle kappa. (B) Schematic ray diagram showing the incident ray passing through the ring edge area in an eye with large angle kappa.

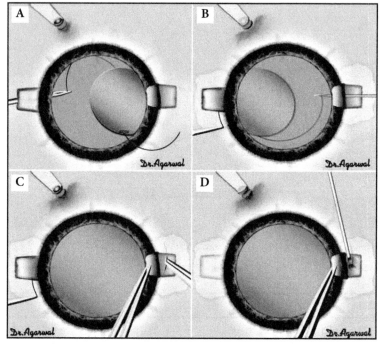

Figure 2-21. Illustration of multifocal glued IOL surgery. (A) Handshake technique. (B) Haptics externalized. (C) Haptic tucked. (D) Fibrin glue applied. (Reprinted with permission from Agarwal A, Jacob S. *Illustrative Guide to Cataract Surgery: A Step-by-Step Approach to Refining Surgical Skills.* Thorofare, NJ: SLACK Incorporated; 2011.)

MULTIFOCAL THREE-PIECE GLUED IOL

There are certain situations in which, despite the best attempts, a centered multifocal IOL in the bag may not be possible in a patient who wants a multifocal lens. In such a patient, it is possible to perform the glued IOL technique and to adjust the centration by adjusting the location of the scleral flaps, sclerotomies, and the degree of tuck of individual haptics. In other situations, such as microspherophakia, our preference is to perform a lensectomy and implant a glued IOL (which must be centered on its rings if it is multifocal). It would also be ideal to combine this with ray optics and center the IOL so that the light ray passes from fixation through the center of the rings to the fovea. A 3-piece multifocal IOL should be used for this (Figure 2-21). Abbott Medical Optics (AMO) is the one company at present that has a 3-piece multifocal IOL.

In the event of a PC rent, it is not advisable to place a multifocal IOL in the sulcus for fear of postoperative decentration. If an in-the-bag multifocal IOL is not possible, a glued multifocal IOL may be preferable because the IOL is very stable and has no postoperative decentration of the IOL occurring from its intraoperative positioning. In all these complicated situations and in patients undergoing routine multifocal lens implantation, it is important to take the angle kappa into consideration for IOL centration. Future advances may also include IOL customization to match the angle kappa of the patients, although postoperative capsular contraction and IOL rotation would be challenges to overcome.

For a multifocal glued IOL, we use an AMO 3-piece lens. When using this IOL, the surgeon is able to tuck the haptics to the point at which the IOL is well centered.

MICROCORNEA

Eyes with microcornea benefit from a glued IOL.[10] Imagine an eye with a white-to-white diameter of 8 mm. If a standard 12-mm foldable IOL is used in this eye, it will be crumpled in the bag. In the glued IOL technique, the haptics are externalized so that only the 6-mm optic is in the eye. The extra bit of haptic that is not needed for the tuck can be cut with scissors. The one problem in microcornea is that we cannot operate on eyes with a white-to-white diameter of less than 7 mm because the IOL optic is 6 mm. For such small eyes, one may have to design a new IOL with smaller optic.

REFERENCES

1. Chan CK, Agarwal A, Agarwal S, Agarwal A. Management of dislocated intraocular implants. *Ophthalmol Clin North Am.* 2001;14(4):681-693.
2. Maggi R, Maggi C. Sutureless scleral fixation of intraocular lenses. *J Cataract Refract Surg.* 1997;23(9):1289-1294.
3. Gabor SG, Pavilidis MM. Sutureless intrascleral posterior chamber intraocular lens fixation. *J Cataract Refract Surg.* 2007;33(11):1851-1854.
4. Agarwal A, Kumar DA, Jacob S, Baid C, Agarwal A, Srinivasan S. Fibrin glue-assisted sutureless posterior chamber intraocular lens implantation in eyes with deficient posterior capsules. *J Cataract Refract Surg.* 2008;34(9):1433-1438.
5. Prakash G, Ashokumar D, Jacob S, Kumar KS, Agarwal A, Agarwal A. Anterior segment optical coherence tomography aided diagnosis and primary posterior chamber intraocular lens implantation with fibrin glue in traumatic phacocele with scleral perforation. *J Cataract Refract Surg.* 2009;35(4):782-784.

6.   Nair V, Kumar DA, Prakash G, Jacob S, Agarwal A, Agarwal A. Bilateral spontaneous in-the-bag anterior subluxation of PC IOL managed with glued IOL technique: a case report. *Eye Contact Lens.* 2009;35(4):215-217.

7.   Kumar DA, Agarwal A, Jacob S, Prakash G, Agarwal A, Sivagnanam S. Repositioning of the dislocated intraocular lens with sutureless 20-gauge vitrectomy. *Retina.* 2010;30(4):682-687.

8.   Prakash G, Agarwal A, Kumar DA, Saleem A, Jacob S, Agarwal A. Translocation of malpositioned posterior chamber intraocular lens from anterior to posterior chamber along with fibrin glue-assisted transscleral fixation. *Eye Contact Lens.* 2010;36(1):45-48.

9.   Ashok Kumar D, Agarwal A, Sivangnanam S, Chandrasekar R, Agarwal A. Implantation of glued intraocular lenses in eyes with microcornea. *J Cataract Refract Surg.* 2015;41(2):327-333.

10. Jacob S, Agarwal A, Agarwal A, Agarwal A, Narasimhan S, Ashok Kumar D. Glued capsular hook: technique for fibrin glue-assisted sutureless transscleral fixation of the capsular bag in subluxated cataracts and intraocular lenses. *J Cataract Refract Surg.* 2014;40(12):1958-1965.

11. Jacob S, Agarwal A. Fibrin glue assisted trans-scleral fixation of an endocapsular device for sutureless trans-scleral capsular bag fixation in traumatic subluxations: the glued endocapsular ring/segment. *Med Hypothesis Discov Innov Ophthalmol.* 2013;2(1):3-7.

12. Ashok Kumar D, Agarwal A, Agarwal A, Chandrasekar R. Clinical outcomes of glued transscleral fixated intraocular lens in functionally one-eyed patients. *Eye Contact Lens.* 2014;40(4):e23-e28.

13. Agarwal A, Narang P, Agarwal A, Kumar DA. Sleeveless-extrusion cannula for levitation of dislocated intraocular lens. *Br J Ophthalmol.* 2014;98(7):910-914.

14. Kumar DA, Agarwal A, Jacob S, Lamba M, Packialakshmi S, Meduri A. Combined surgical management of capsular and iris deficiency with glued intraocular lens technique. *J Refract Surg.* 2013;29(5):342-347.

15. Kumar DA, Agarwal A, Prakash G, Jacob S. Managing total aniridia with aphakia using a glued iris prosthesis. *J Cataract Refract Surg.* 2010;36(5):864-865.

16. Agarwal A, Jacob S, Kumar DA, Agarwal A, Narasimhan S, Agarwal A. Handshake technique for glued intrascleral haptic fixation of a posterior chamber intraocular lens. *J Cataract Refract Surg.* 2013;39(3):317-322.

17. Kumar DA, Agarwal A, Prakash D, Prakash G, Jacob S, Agarwal A. Glued intrascleral fixation of posterior chamber intraocular lens in children. *Am J Ophthalmol.* 2012;153(4):594-601.

18. Prakash G, Agarwal A, Prakash DR, Kumar DA, Agarwal A, Jacob S. Role of angle kappa in patient dissatisfaction with refractive-design multifocal intraocular lenses. *J Cataract Refract Surg.* 2011;37(9):1739-1740.

19. Gooi P, Teichman JC, Ahmed II. Sutureless intrascleral fixation of a custom-tailored iris prosthesis with an intraocular lens. *J Cataract Refract Surg.* 2014;40(11):1759-1763.

3

Glued IOL
Scaffold Procedure
Managing Nuclear
Fragments in Eyes With
Deficient Posterior Capsule

Priya Narang, MS and
Amar Agarwal, MS, FRCS, FRCOphth

The word *scaffold* is derived from the Latin word *scaffaldus* meaning "a temporary platform." As the name suggests, the glued intraocular lens (IOL) scaffold[1] is a technique that combines 2 major techniques: glued intrascleral haptic fixation of IOL (glued IOL)[2] and IOL scaffold.[3,4] Glued IOL is a type of secondary IOL fixation, whereas IOL scaffold (Figures 3-1 and 3-2) is a surgical technique described for facilitating nucleus emulsification in cases of inadvertent posterior capsule rupture (PCR). In PCR, the nuclear fragments are levitated into the anterior chamber (AC), and an IOL is preplaced either in the sulcus or above the iris, followed by subsequent introduction of the phacoemulsification probe into the eye to emulsify the nuclear fragments (Figure 3-3). PCR in association with nonemulsified nuclear fragments and an absent sulcus support is a challenging scenario for the anterior segment surgeon. Under such circumstances, the glued IOL scaffold technique helps the surgeon overcome all the limitations, although it calls for specific surgical skills.

Agarwal A, ed.
A Video Textbook of Glued IOLs (pp 61-74).
© 2016 Taylor & Francis Group.

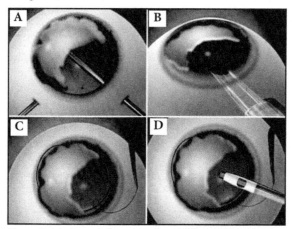

Figure 3-1. Animated demonstration of IOL scaffold. (A) Nuclear remnants lifted into the AC. (B) A 3-piece foldable IOL injected beneath the nuclear remnant. (C) Trailing haptic left extruded from the corneal incision. Both haptics can be placed above the iris or above the rhexis also. (D) Phacoemulsification probe introduced above the IOL.

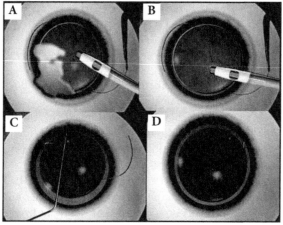

Figure 3-2. Animated demonstration of IOL scaffold. (A) Nuclear remnants being emulsified. (B) Phacoemulsification complete. (C) IOL being dialed into sulcus. One can dilate the pupil with iris hooks at this stage once the nucleus is removed to assess the amount of capsule present and depending on the amount of capsule present one can put the 3-piece IOL in the sulcus or make it a glued IOL. (D) Well-placed IOL above capsulorrhexis.

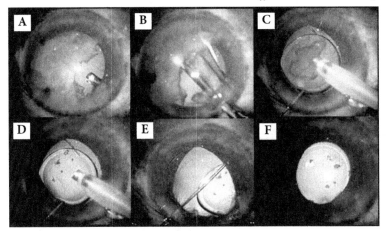

Figure 3-3. Surgical steps of IOL scaffold. (A) Nuclear fragments are levitated into the anterior chamber and vitrectomy is performed. (B) Two partial scleral thickness scleral flaps are made 180 degrees opposite each other followed by sclerotomy. A 3-piece foldable IOL is injected beneath the nuclear fragments. (C) Haptics of the IOL placed on the anterior surface of iris tissue. Emulsification of the nuclear fragment is performed with a phacoemulsification probe. (D) Nuclear fragments are emulsified. (E) IOL is dialed onto the sulcus support. (F) A well-placed and centered IOL.

Preplacement and prefixation of an IOL by using the glued IOL scaffold (Figure 3-4) method effectively compartmentalizes the AC and PC. The preplaced IOL acts as an artificial PC and enables safe emulsification of the nuclear fragments. Depending on the accessibility to instruments and surgeon comfort, a retinal surgeon may manage the subluxed crystalline or dislocated IOL.

SURGICAL PROCEDURE

After an intraoperative PCR, the surgery is temporarily halted and viscoelastic is injected from the sideport incision before withdrawal of the phacoemulsification probe from the eye. As in a glued IOL surgery, 2 partial-thickness scleral flaps are made 180 degrees opposite each other (Figure 3-5A). Sclerotomy is done with a 20-gauge needle approximately 1.5 mm away from the limbus, beneath the scleral flaps. The nucleus/nuclear fragments are levitated and brought into the AC with the help of the posterior assisted levitation (PAL) technique (Figure 3-5B). Infusion is introduced into the eye with the help of either a trocar cannula or a trocar

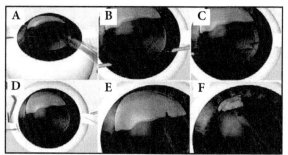

Figure 3-4. Animated demonstration of the glued IOL scaffold technique. Intraoperative PCR is noted. Nuclear pieces are brought to the AC. (A) Vitrectomy is done. A 3-piece foldable IOL is implanted. Note the cartridge in the AC. Also note that the haptic is slightly out of the cartridge so that it is easy for the glued IOL forceps to grasp the tip of the haptic with the handshake technique; (B) Haptics are transferred from one glued IOL forceps to another. (C) Handshake technique completed. (D) Both haptics are externalized and tucked in Scharioth pocket. (E) Phacoemulsion of the nuclear pieces. Artificial posterior capsule created by the IOL. (F) Nucleus emulsified. Note that the IOL scaffold and the glued IOL procedure combined prevent the nucleus from falling down. Nucleus totally emulsified.

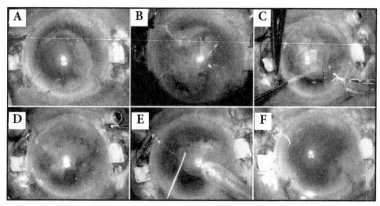

Figure 3-5. Surgical steps of glued IOL scaffold after posterior assisted levitation (PAL). (A) Posterior capsule rupture with nonemulsified nucleus. (B) Nuclear fragments levitated into the anterior chamber with PAL. (C) A 3-piece foldable IOL is injected beneath the nucleus fragment and glued IOL procedure is performed. Leading haptic of the IOL is externalized. (D) Trailing haptic is maneuvered inside the eye and externalized. (E) Haptics tucked in to the scleral pockets. Phacoemulsification probe introduced into the eye and the nuclear fragments are emulsified as in an IOL scaffold procedure. (F) Corneal wound secured with 10-0 suture. Stromal hydration is performed.

AC maintainer. Care is taken to direct the flow of fluid in a way that it does not dislodge the nuclear fragments into the vitreous cavity. A 23-gauge vitrectomy cutter is introduced from the sclerotomy site and from the corneal tunnel incision to enable a thorough vitrectomy to be performed in the pupillary plane. A 3-piece foldable IOL is loaded and injected beneath the nuclear fragments and the tip of the leading haptic is grasped with glued IOL forceps. When the entire IOL has unfolded, the tip of the leading haptic is pulled and externalized (Figure 3-5C). The trailing haptic is then flexed into the eye, and the handshake technique is performed for its externalization. The externalized haptics (Figure 3-5D) are then tucked into the scleral pockets created with a 26-gauge needle.

After tucking of the haptics, the pupil is narrowed down with the help of pilocarpine to prevent any accidental dislodgement of the nuclear fragments from around the edges of the IOL. The phacoemulsification probe is then introduced, and the nuclear fragments are emulsified (Figure 3-5E). The corneal wound is secured with a 10-0 suture, stromal hydration is performed to seal all the corneal wounds (Figure 3-5F), and air is injected into the AC. Fibrin glue is applied beneath the scleral flaps and along the conjunctival peritomy incision.

This technique has been applied in varied scenarios, such as dropped nucleus,[5] subluxation of lens,[6] and for Soemmering ring removal when associated with a deficient posterior capsule.[7]

ROLE OF POSTERIOR ASSISTED LEVITATION TECHNIQUE IN GLUED IOL SCAFFOLD

The PAL technique[8] enables levitation of the nucleus/nuclear fragments from the anterior vitreous into the AC. This procedure can be done with the assistance of a rod/blunt spatula (see Figure 3-5B) or with the help of the injection of viscoelastic,[9] which forms a base below the nuclear fragments and prevents them from further dislodgement into the vitreous cavity.

When beginning PAL, a sclerotomy wound is created with the help of either a microvitreoretinal (MVR) blade or a trocar cannula (depending on the surgeon's preference) approximately 3 to 3.5 mm from the limbus. The MVR blade is directed obliquely toward the midvitreous cavity. A blunt rod or spatula is inserted from the sclerotomy site, and the nucleus/nuclear fragment is supported at its base and then levitated into the AC. It is advisable to place the levitated fragments onto the anterior surface of the iris along

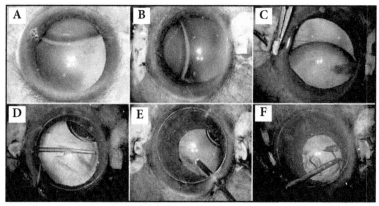

Figure 3-6. Surgical steps of glued IOL scaffold procedure for traumatic subluxated cataract. (A) Traumatic subluxation of the lens. (B) The surgeon sits temporally and 2 partial-thickness scleral flaps are made 180 degrees opposite each other at the 6 o'clock and 12 o'clock positions. (C) Sclerotomy done with a 20-gauge needle approximately 1.5 mm from the limbus, beneath the scleral flaps. (D) The subluxated lens is lifted with the help of a rod (PAL) introduced from the sclerotomy site. The lens is lifted and is placed into the AC. Pilocarpine is injected into the AC to constrict the pupil. (E) Vitrectomy is performed beneath the lens to cut down all vitreous adhesions. (F) A 3-piece foldable IOL is loaded and injected beneath the subluxated lens, and the leading haptic is externalized, followed by the trailing haptic. The handshake technique is performed for externalization of the trailing haptic beneath the lens.

the AC angle so that they do not slip back into the vitreous cavity. Some surgeons prefer using viscoelastic for nucleus levitation, although the use of viscoelastic in the vitreous cavity should be curtailed because retained viscoelastic often can lead to inflammation.

GLUED IOL SCAFFOLD FOR TRAUMATIC SUBLUXATED LENS

In cases of traumatic subluxated lens,[6] PAL is performed initially, and the entire nucleus is levitated into the AC; it is then made to rest on the anterior surface of the iris. The glued IOL scaffold is eventually performed, and the entire nucleus is subsequently emulsified (Figures 3-6 and 3-7).

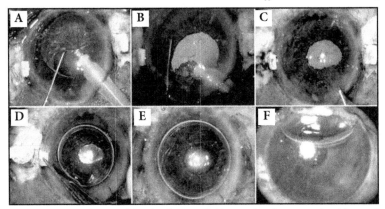

Figure 3-7. Surgical steps of the glued IOL scaffold procedure for traumatic subluxated cataract. (A) IOL fixed beneath the lens by glued IOL technique now acts as a scaffold. The crystalline lens is then emulsified with the phacoemulsification probe. (B) Nuclear emulsification nearly completed. (C) The corneal wound is secured with a 10-0 nylon suture. (D) Fibrin glue is applied beneath the flaps. (E) The scleral flaps and conjunctival peritomy are sealed with fibrin glue. (F) The patient on the first postoperative day.

GLUED IOL SCAFFOLD PROCEDURE FOR SOEMMERING RING WITH ASSOCIATED POSTERIOR CAPSULE RUPTURE

Various techniques have been described in peer-reviewed literature for managing Soemmering ring and subsequent IOL implantation. It is very tricky to handle Soemmering ring when it is associated with a PCR. The glued IOL scaffold procedure can be implemented in such a scenario.[7]

Soemmering ring has a typical peripheral disposition (Figure 3-8A) and it is usually present around the peripheral edges of the pupillary margin. Vitrectomy is performed around the margins of Soemmering ring so the Soemmering material is not disrupted (Figure 3-8B). A 3-piece foldable IOL is introduced (Figure 3-8C), and the glued IOL procedure is performed (Figures 3-8D through F).

Preplacement of an IOL by using the glued IOL scaffold technique helps to form a base for the Soemmering ring. After fixation of an IOL by the glued IOL method, vitrectomy is performed around the periphery of the Soemmering ring to release all the vitreous strands and adhesions. In cases of small pupil, iris hooks are used to visualize the Soemmering ring clearly

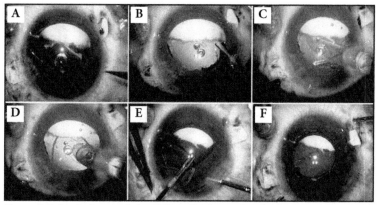

Figure 3-8. Surgical steps of glued IOL scaffold procedure for Soemmering ring with associated PCR (part 1). (A) Soemmering ring present in the periphery. (B) Vitrectomy is performed to cut down vitreous adhesions surrounding the ring. (C) A 3-piece fold-able IOL is injected beneath the Soemmering ring. The tip of the haptic is grasped with glued IOL forceps. (D) Slow unfolding of the IOL. (E) The leading haptic is pulled and externalized. The trailing haptic is flexed into the eye. (F) Both haptics are externalized. (Reprinted with permission from Agarwal A. Glued intraocular lens scaffolding for Soemmering ring removal in aphakia with posterior capsule defect. *J Cataract Refract Surg.* 2015;41[4]:703-718.)

(Figure 3-9A). The Soemmering ring is then dislodged with a dialer and is brought into the center of the pupil (Figures 3-9B and C). In cases of widely dilated pupil, the pupil is constricted with an intraocular miotic agent to prevent any inadvertent loss of Soemmering ring material from around the peripheral edges of the IOL into the vitreous cavity. In cases in which iris hooks were used for adequate visualization, the iris hooks are removed for the same reason (Figure 3-9D). Phacoemulsification is then performed (Figure 3-9E), and the Soemmering material is eventually emulsified (Figure 3-9F). The scleral flaps are then sealed with fibrin glue and the corneal wound is secured with a 10-0 suture (Figure 3-10).

GLUED IOL SCAFFOLD PROCEDURE FOR DROPPED NUCLEUS

For management of cases that are associated with dropped nucleus and inadequate sulcus support, a combination of glued IOL scaffold with sleeve-less phacotip assisted levitation (SPAL)[5] is employed. SPAL is a technique

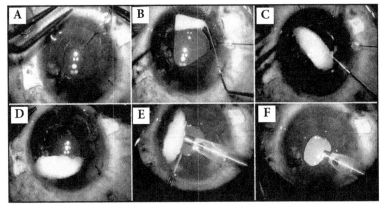

Figure 3-9. Surgical steps of the glued IOL scaffold procedure for Soemmering ring with associated PCR (part 2). (A) Iris hooks being introduced into the eye. (B) Soemmering ring is dislodged from the periphery with the help of dialer. (C) Soemmering ring dislodged in the center. (D) Iris hooks are removed to prevent any accidental dislodgement of Soemmering ring material from the peripheral edges of the IOL. (E) Soemmering ring being emulsified with the phacoemulsification probe. (F) All of the Soemmering material is emulsified. A well-centered and well-placed IOL is seen. (Reprinted with permission from Agarwal A. Glued intraocular lens scaffolding for Soemmering ring removal in aphakia with posterior capsule defect. *J Cataract Refract Surg.* 2015;41[4]:703-718.)

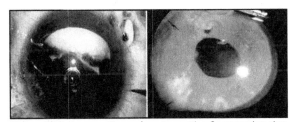

Figure 3-10. Preoperative and postoperative Soemmering ring after the glued IOL scaffold procedure. (Reprinted with permission from Agarwal A. Glued intraocular lens scaffolding for Soemmering ring removal in aphakia with posterior capsule defect. *J Cataract Refract Surg.* 2015;41[4]:703-718.)

that facilitates the levitation of dropped nucleus (Figure 3-11A) into the AC. SPAL eliminates the need to emulsify the nucleus in the vitreous cavity and its subsequent complications. Holding the nucleus with a sleeveless phacotip enables a firm grip, keeping the nucleus from falling back into the vitreous cavity (Figure 3-12). The firmly embedded nucleus is then easy to levitate into the AC. The recommended technique for using ultrasound energy in the vitreous cavity is to lift the nucleus fragment away from the retinal

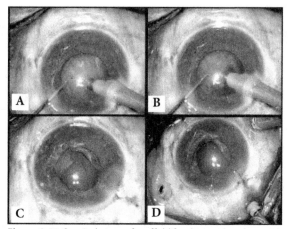

Figure 3-11. Surgical steps of scaffold for dropped nucleus with SPAL procedure (part 1). (A) Phacoemulsification is performed. (B) Posterior capsule rupture. (C) Dropped nucleus. (D) Standard 3-port pars plana vitrectomy incisions framed.

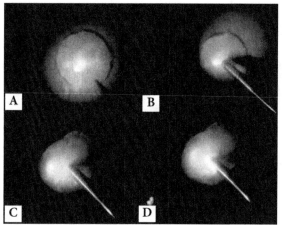

Figure 3-12. Surgical steps of the scaffold procedure for dropped nucleus with SPAL (part 2). (A) Vitrectomy is performed and all adhesions surrounding the dropped nucleus are removed. (B) Sleeveless phacotip is introduced and brought near the dropped fragment. (C) The dropped nucleus is lifted from the surface of the retina into the vitreous cavity. (D) The nucleus is embedded with a short burst of phaco power, which prevents the nucleus from falling back onto the surface of the retina.

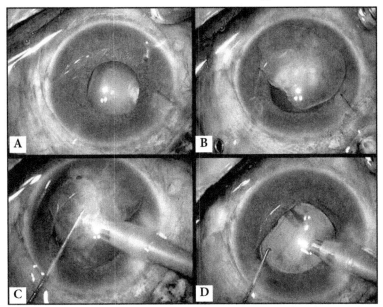

Figure 3-13. Surgical steps of the scaffold procedure for dropped nucleus with SPAL (part 3). (A) The nucleus is levitated and brought into the pupillary plane. (B) The nucleus is manipulated into the AC. (C) A 3-piece foldable IOL is injected beneath the nucleus and placed into the sulcus. The nuclear fragment is emulsified. (D) Nucleus emulsification is complete.

surface by aspiration in the mid/anterior vitreous cavity, thereby limiting exposure of the posterior pole to ultrasound energy.

Once the nucleus is levitated into the AC (Figures 3-13A and B), a glued IOL scaffold procedure is performed in cases of inadequate sulcus support, although, in cases with adequate sulcus support, an IOL scaffold procedure (Figures 3-13C and D) will suffice.

DISCUSSION

Glued IOL scaffold (Figures 3-14 and 3-15) is an excellent procedure that allows closed chamber manipulation with simultaneous implantation of the IOL. This technique requires proper handling and management of disturbed vitreous and the nuclear fragments. It also requires the surgeon to be very well versed in the principles of vitrectomy and glued IOL surgery.

The size of the pupil plays a significant role in this procedure. We recommend having a wide pupil during nucleus levitation into the AC. Iris

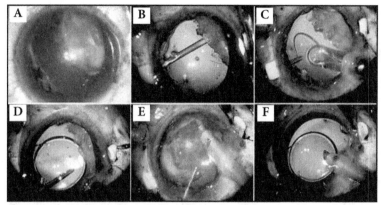

Figure 3-14. The glued IOL scaffold procedure for a traumatic subluxated cataract. (A) Traumatic subluxated cataract. (B) Vitrectomy. (C) Glued IOL scaffold. (D) Haptics externalized. (E) Phacoemulsification done. Notice that the cataract is brought anterior to the IOL. (F) Phacoemulsification completed.

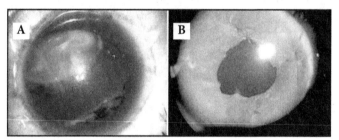

Figure 3-15. Preoperative and postoperative images. (A) Preoperative image of a patient with traumatic subluxated lens. (B) Postoperative image of the same patient 1 month later.

hooks, if needed, are often employed for this. Following the fixation of the IOL, the pupil is constricted with an intraocular miotic agent or by removal of iris hooks. Constricting the pupil at this stage prevents any inadvertent dislodgement of the nuclear fragment into the vitreous cavity from around the edges of the IOL.

In the IOL scaffold procedure, the IOL is placed on either the sulcus support or on the anterior surface of the iris, followed by emulsification with the help of a phacoemulsification probe. It cannot be performed if the iris or sulcus support is inadequate. Glued IOL scaffold comes to the rescue because it can be performed in such a scenario. The preplaced IOL acts as a scaffold or as an artificial PC and facilitates emulsification of the fragments. In addition, the glued IOL scaffold technique allows prefixing of the IOL in its normal anatomical position in the PC. As a result, adequate depth of the AC is available for the complete emulsification of the nuclear material. Adequate coating of the endothelium with a dispersive ophthalmic viscosurgical device is recommended to protect the endothelium. Adequate infusion into the eye also helps to stabilize the AC and maintain the integrity of the globe during surgery.

This technique is applicable in cases of traumatic subluxation of the lens and also in Soemmering ring management with associated PC dehiscence. In cases of traumatic subluxation of the lens or dropped nucleus, the entire lens is elevated into the AC, and the technique is performed. It is essential to note that proficiency in glued IOL surgery is a must in cases of hard and large nuclei that often occupy the entire AC because the handshake technique[10] must be performed for externalization of the haptics that lie beneath the hard nucleus. Moreover, because visualization of the IOL is impaired, it is crucial for the surgeon to perform the handshake technique with tactile sensation of the feel of haptics.

This technique is not recommended for dense, brown cataracts because it can often lead to decompensation of the endothelium. Under such circumstances, extracapsular cataract extraction can be performed to optimize the visual outcome and prevent any inadvertent damage to the endothelium.

CONCLUSION

The glued IOL scaffold serves as an effective method with good postoperative results (see Figure 3-15) for select cases of complicated cataract surgery with associated PCR and inadequate sulcus or iris support.

REFERENCES

1. Agarwal A, Jacob S, Agarwal A, Narasimhan S, Kumar DA, Agarwal A. Glued intraocular lens scaffolding to create an artificial posterior capsule for nucleus removal in eyes with posterior capsule tear and insufficient iris and sulcus support. *J Cataract Refract Surg.* 2013;39(3):326-333.
2. Agarwal A, Kumar DA, Jacob S, Baid C, Agarwal A, Srinivasan S. Fibrin glue-assisted sutureless posterior chamber intraocular lens implantation in eyes with deficient posterior capsules. *J Cataract Refract Surg.* 2008;34(9):1433-1438.
3. Kumar DA, Agarwal A, Prakash G, Jacob S, Agarwal A, Sivagnanam S. IOL scaffold technique for posterior capsule rupture [letter]. *J Refract Surg.* 2012;28(5):314-315.

4. Narang P, Agarwal A, Kumar DA, Jacob S, Agarwal A, Agarwal A. Clinical outcomes of intraocular lens scaffold surgery. A one-year study. *Ophthalmology.* 2013;120(12):2442-2448.

5. Agarwal A, Narang P, A Kumar D, Agarwal A. Clinical outcomes of sleeveless phacotip assisted levitation of dropped nucleus. *Br J Ophthalmol.* 2014;98(10):1429-1434.

6. Narang P, Agarwal A, Kumar DA, Agarwal A. Clinical outcomes of the glued intraocular lens scaffold. *J Cataract Refract Surg.* 2015;41(9):1867-1874.

7. Narang P, Agarwal A, Kumar DA. Glued intraocular lens scaffolding for Soemmerring ring removal in aphakia with posterior capsule defect. *J Cataract Refract Surg.* 2015;41(4):708-713.

8. Packard RBS, Kinnear FC. *Manual of Cataract and Intraocular Lens Surgery.* Edinburgh, United Kingdom: Churchill Livingstone;1991:47.

9. Chang DF, Packard RB. Posterior assisted levitation for nucleus retrieval using Viscoat after posterior capsule rupture. *J Cataract Refract Surg.* 2003;29(10):1860-1865.

10. Agarwal A, Jacob S, Kumar DA, Agarwal A, Narsimhan S, Agarwal A. Handshake technique for glued intrascleral fixation of a posterior chamber intraocular lens. *J Cataract Refract Surg.* 2013;39(3):317-322.

4

Corneal Surgery With Glued IOL, Including Pre-Descemet's Endothelial Keratoplasty

Soosan Jacob, MS, FRCS, Dip NB
and Amar Agarwal MS, FRCS, FRCOphth

The glued intraocular lens (IOL) was introduced in 2007 as a technique for sutureless scleral fixation of the IOL via transscleral haptic tuck in patients with absent or deficient capsular support.[1-13] This technique may be used as a primary procedure during cataract extraction in cases of posterior capsular rupture (PCR) and deficient capsule or as a secondary procedure in a patient with aphasia. It also may be used for closed-chamber translocation of a malpositioned or subluxated 3-piece IOL. However, many of these patients who need primary or secondary glued IOL implantation have already undergone complicated cataract surgery in which the surgeon was unable to implant an IOL in the bag during the cataract extraction. Therefore, the chances of endothelial damage and the consequent need for a keratoplasty are also higher in these patients. Depending on the severity of endothelial damage and corneal scarring, the patient may require either a penetrating keratoplasty (PK) or an endothelial keratoplasty (EK).

Agarwal A, ed.
A Video Textbook of Glued IOLs (pp 75-98).
© 2016 Taylor & Francis Group.

GLUED IOL WITH PENETRATING KERATOPLASTY

Glued IOL may be combined with a penetrating keratoplasty (PK) when there is associated stromal scarring. The PK can be performed with the help of a femtosecond laser (Figures 4-1 through 4-4). The advantages of glued IOL with PK over other forms of secondary IOL fixation are the relatively short open sky time and the sturdy fixation of the IOL.

Technique

If the white-to-white diameter is more than 11.5 to 12 mm, a vertical glued IOL may be used to get more haptic exteriorized for the intrascleral tuck. Conjunctival peritomy and partial-thickness scleral flaps are made 180 degrees opposite each other. Partial-thickness trephination of the recipient cornea is performed, followed by 20-gauge sclerotomies under the scleral flaps. The intrascleral Scharioth tunnels are created in line with the sclerotomy. The creation of the flaps, the sclerotomies, and the Scharioth tunnels are easier with a closed globe; therefore, the anterior chamber (AC) is entered only after these steps have been completed. A sideport knife is then used to enter the AC through the partial-thickness trephine, and the recipient cornea is excised along the trephined groove. Any vitreous in the AC is cleared with a vitrector. Microforceps are introduced through the 20-gauge sclerotomy, and the leading haptic of the 3-piece IOL is grasped and exteriorized through the 20-gauge sclerotomy on the left side. This is followed by similarly exteriorizing the trailing haptic on the right side. Because this is an open-sky procedure, the exteriorization is easy and must be done quickly in order to decrease open sky time. While introducing the microforceps through the 20-gauge sclerotomy, care is taken to enter atraumatically, avoiding any pushing of the choroid because the risk of choroidal detachment is higher in open sky procedures. Once both the haptics have been exteriorized, the IOL is generally stable and does not show a tendency to drop. The haptics may now be tucked into the intrascleral tunnels, although tucking is more difficult in a hypotonic state. Alternatively, if an adequate length of exteriorized haptic has been obtained, the haptics may be left outside and untucked until 8 sutures have been applied. The surgeon must keep an eye on the haptics at all times to avoid any slippage. The haptics may also be secured with Serafano clips to prevent slippage. The donor corneal graft is then sutured in place. Once the graft is sutured, the haptics may be tucked into the intrascleral Scharioth tunnels with greater ease. Vitrectomy is performed under the scleral flaps, and the flaps and

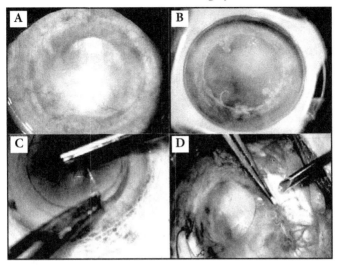

Figure 4-1. Femtosecond laser-assisted PK with glued IOL (part 1). (A) Preoperative photograph showing pseudophakic bullous keratopathy (PBK) with an AC IOL in situ. (B) Femtosecond laser-created top-hat configuration. (C) Femtosecond-assisted top-hat configuration showing predictable and uniform wound formation. (D) Inferior straight sclerotomy made with a 20-gauge needle 1.5 mm from the limbus under the existing scleral flaps. Note the diametrically opposite scleral flaps. (Reprinted with permission from Agarwal A, Femtosecond-assisted keratoplasty with fibrin glue-assisted sutureless posterior chamber lens implantation: new triple procedure. *J Cataract Refract Surg.* 2009;35[6]:973-979.)

conjunctiva are stuck with fibrin glue. Balanced salt solution is injected gently into the AC after loosening the speculum to make sure that the globe is not left hypotonic in the end.

Femto-Assisted Keratoplasty With Glued IOL

We have performed femtosecond laser-assisted PK with AC IOL explantation and glued IOL (see Figures 4-1 through 4-4) and documented it in a peer-reviewed journal.[14] Creation of the donor and host corneal button is achieved with a femtosecond laser. Donor buttons are prepared from whole globes after application of the suction ring. Adequate vacuum and centration are achieved and a top-hat configuration is created using the IntraLase FS femtosecond laser (IntraLase Corp). For the host cut, topical anesthetic agent is instilled into the patient's eye. The suction ring

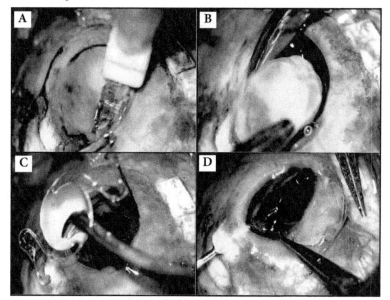

Figure 4-2. Femtosecond laser-assisted PK with glued IOL (part 2). (A) Augmentation of the top-hat configuration in areas that had poor laser penetration because of overlying opacity. (B) Posterior uncut tissue dissected with Vannas scissors. (C) Explantation of an AC IOL after removal of the host button. (D) Leading haptic grasped with the microcapsulorrhexis forceps for being pulled through the inferior sclerotomy following the haptic curve. (Reprinted with permission from Agarwal A. Femtosecond-assisted keratoplasty with fibrin glue-assisted sutureless posterior chamber lens implantation: new triple procedure. *J Cataract Refract Surg.* 2009;35[6]973-979.)

is similarly applied, and after adequate vacuum and centration, a top-hat configuration is created.

The donor corneal tissue and patient are then taken to the keratoplasty operating room with the patient and the rest of the surgery is performed with the patient under peribulbar anesthesia. As previously explained, 2 partial-thickness scleral flaps are made, followed by sclerotomy. The top hat is inspected for completeness. After the host button is removed, limited open-sky anterior vitrectomy is performed. The haptics are then externalized, followed by tucking in the scleral pockets. The graft is placed, and cardinal sutures are applied. The reconstituted fibrin glue is injected through the cannula of the syringe delivery system under both the scleral flaps. The same glue can be applied in the area between the sutures at the entire graft–host junction. The conjunctiva is also apposed with the glue.

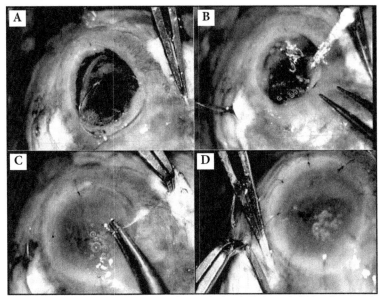

Figure 4-3. Femtosecond laser-assisted PK with glued IOL (part 3). (A) Leading haptic externalized completely under the inferior scleral flap. (B) The trailing haptic externalized through the superior sclerotomy under the scleral flap. (C) The graft button placed and cardinal sutures applied. (D) Scleral tunnel created along the curve of the externalized haptic in the superonasal area at the edge of the scleral bed of the flap. (Reprinted with permission from Agarwal A. Femtosecond-assisted keratoplasty with fibrin glue-assisted sutureless posterior chamber lens implantation: new triple procedure. *J Cataract Refract Surg.* 2009;35[6]:973-979.)

Advantages

The glued IOL can be performed in much less open-sky time than other secondary IOL fixation techniques. Once the haptics have been exteriorized, the optic acts as a tamponade and is helpful in preventing expulsive hemorrhage. It can also be done with any 3-piece IOL available without the need for a special IOL with eyelets on the haptic. The glued IOL procedure may be performed even in hypotonous eyes, and centration can be adjusted once the graft is sutured and the globe is formed. Lack of pseudophacodonesis is another advantage of the glued IOL technique over other secondary IOL-fixation techniques (Figure 4-5).

While performing scleral fixation with sutures, the surgeon must readjust the knots to maintain the central position of the IOL. In our procedure, simply manipulating the amount of externalization can cause proper centration of the IOL. The final tucking of the haptic provides additional

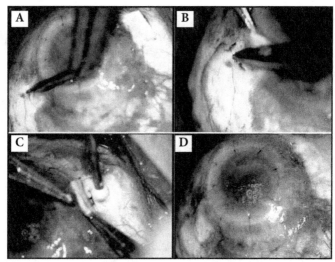

Figure 4-4. Femtosecond laser-assisted PK with glued IOL (part 4). (A) The superior haptic tucked into the superonasal tunnel. (B) The tucking shown at higher magnification. (C) Reconstituted fibrin glue injected through the cannula of the syringe delivery system under the inferior scleral flap. (D) The glue applied at the graft-host junction. (Reprinted with permission from Agarwal A. Femtosecond-assisted keratoplasty with fibrin glue-assisted sutureless posterior chamber lens implantation: new triple procedure. *J Cataract Refract Surg.* 2009;35[6]:973-979.)

stabilization. A sutured sclera-fixated IOL hangs in the posterior chamber, with the sutures passing through the haptic eyes, similar to a hammock, causing dynamic torsional and anteroposterior oscillation. This pseudo-phacodonesis may result in progressive endothelial loss. However, in this technique, haptics are used for fixation on the scleral side, and the stable optic–haptic junction prevents torsional and anteroposterior instability. Therefore, there is much less pseudophacodonesis (see Figure 4-5). The haptics are covered in the scleral flap and tucked well inside the scleral pocket. There is an additional well-apposed layer of conjunctiva over the sclera. This further reduces the chances of haptic extrusion.

Femtosecond laser-assisted keratoplasty with top-hat configuration and a glued IOL provides a unique solution in cases of bullous keratopathy and AC IOLs. This is an improvement over the traditional technique of manual trephination and transscleral suture fixation of the IOL (see Figure 4-5). The femtosecond laser's top-hat configuration provides a greater number of endothelial cells in the donor lenticule and a more stable wound configuration. Better dynamic stability of the glued IOL prevents pseudophacodonesis

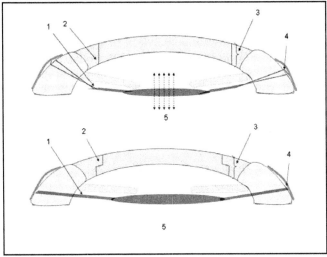

Figure 4-5. Biomechanical and kinetic properties of manual keratoplasty with transscleral suture-fixated posterior capsule (PC) IOL (TSF IOL) (top) and femtosecond laser-assisted keratoplasty with glued IOL (bottom). Differences between the 2 approaches are indicated by the points. Point 1, top: Haptic-suture junction in the TSF IOL, with the IOL hanging like a hammock. Point 1, bottom: Rigid polymethylmethacrylate-haptic in glued IOL fixated with the sclera. Point 2, top: Transverse graft-host junction. Point 2, bottom: More stable top-hat configuration. Point 3, top: Size of epithelial side (outer cut) is the same as that of endothelial side (inner cut). Point 3, bottom: Size of epithelial side (outer cut) less than that of endothelial side (inner cut), leading to a greater number of endothelial cells for smaller epithelial load and placement of sutures farther from the limbus. Point 4, top: Knots in TSF IOL may degrade and slip. Point 4, bottom: Haptic is securely tucked and sealed with fibrin glue in glued IOL. Point 5, top: More pseudophacodonesis with TSF IOL. Point 5, bottom: Less pseudophacodonesis with glued IOL. (Reprinted with permission from Agarwal A. Femtosecond-assisted keratoplasty with fibrin glue-assisted sutureless posterior chamber lens implantation: new triple procedure. *J Cataract Refract Surg.* 2009;35[6]:973-979.)

and may reduce endothelial cell loss or repositioning surgery. Combined, these 2 surgical modalities may improve results.

GLUED IOL WITH ENDOTHELIAL KERATOPLASTY

In patients with predominantly endothelial damage, an endothelial keratoplasty (EK) may be performed instead of a PK. The advantages of

EK include a closed-chamber technique with faster visual recovery, better quality of vision, lesser induction of irregular astigmatism, fewer chances of rejection, and fewer surface- and suture-related problems. There are also likely to be fewer postoperative refractive surprises with EK than with PK. Glued IOL can be combined with Descemet's stripping automated endothelial keratoplasty (DSAEK), Descemet's membrane endothelial keratoplasty (DMEK), or pre-Descemet's endothelial keratoplasty (PDEK). It may also be done as a staged procedure, in which the glued IOL is performed first, and the EK is performed in a second sitting.

Principles of Combining Glued IOL With Endothelial Keratoplasty

In aphakic eyes, a loss of bicamerality of the eye occurs, which leads to posterior migration of the air bubble used for attaching the DMEK graft. This increases the risk for a consequent postoperative partial or total graft detachment, forward bowing of the iris, iris-graft touch, graft dislocation into the vitreous, and so on—all of which can necessitate secondary procedures such as refloating, rebubbling, vitrectomy, and AC formation, which in turn increases graft endothelial cell loss. An effective compartmentalization of the eye can be obtained through the glued IOL technique. The glued IOL offers advantages, including PC IOL placement, ease of centration, and scleral fixation, as well as stable and sturdy fixation without pseudophacodonesis. In contrast, AC IOL has the disadvantages of decreased AC space and iris-fixated IOLs that require intact iris all around. Sutured sclera-fixated IOLs share the disadvantages of greater pseudophacodonesis and greater difficulty in centration.

The procedure is started as a conventional glued IOL. An AC maintainer is inserted. Conjunctival flaps and lamellar scleral flaps are made 180 degrees apart, as explained earlier. Twenty-gauge sclerotomies are made under the scleral flap approximately 1 mm from the limbus. This is followed by limited 23-gauge vitrectomy through the sclerotomies, followed by glued IOL implantation. The haptics are tucked in and the flaps may be glued down. Because the PC is unlikely to be intact, there is still a chance of posterior migration of air that is injected into the AC for graft support. Migration of air behind the IOL leads to insufficient support for the graft, with consequent graft detachment. It is imperative to have a good iris-IOL diaphragm separating the AC from the vitreous cavity. When combining a glued IOL with EK, the sclerotomy should be made slightly closer to the limbus than usual to decrease the potential gap between the iris and the IOL. At the same time, an iridoplasty should be performed to obtain a round pupil that overlaps the IOL optic all around. Once this is done, the infusion is turned off and the adequacy of air fill is checked. If inadequate, the pupil may need to become smaller or the IOL may need to come closer to the iris. A well-formed iris-IOL diaphragm prevents air from going back into the vitreous cavity and provides good postoperative support for the graft. Once the air fill is found to be adequate, air is attached to the AC maintainer through an air pump, and host descemetorhexis is performed. A small inferior peripheral iridotomy is made. The EK graft is then injected into the AC, unfolded, and floated up using air. In extensively vitrectomized eyes, nonexpansile concentration of C3F8 or SF6 may be used instead. Intraocular pressure and light perception are checked, and the patient is advised to lie in the supine position for 24 hours.

In cases with a subluxated or dislocated 3-piece IOL needing EK, a closed-chamber translocation of the subluxated IOL into a glued IOL may be done using the handshake technique. This is followed by iridoplasty (if required) and EK.

Cases with a malpositioned single-piece IOL requiring explantation or an AC IOL need an enlargement of the wound followed by explantation of the IOL. This is followed by the technique described previously. Construction of a scleral tunnel for IOL explantation enables very good wound closure and excellent AC stability.

A potential complication that may occur when combining glued IOL with DMEK is the risk for hypotony and subsequent graft detachment in the postoperative period. Hypotony can lead to detachment of the DMEK graft from the eyelids pushing on the cornea with normal lid movements. This risk can be decreased by ensuring that the globe is adequately pressurized at the end of surgery. As noted, this is done by achieving an adequately tight air bubble in the AC. If the globe still feels hypotonic, balanced salt solution is injected through the pars plicata into the vitreous cavity with a 30-gauge needle under direct visualization of the needle tip in the vitreous cavity. At the conclusion of surgery, the surgeon must also ensure that the sclerotomies are well sealed by the scleral flaps using fibrin glue. All corneal incisions should be leak-proof and may also be sealed using fibrin glue to avoid any postoperative leak of aqueous fluid or escape of air, which could increase the risk of detachment. Patients undergoing the procedure need to be watched more closely after surgery for any evidence of partial or total graft detachments and taken for rebubbling if necessary.

A properly positioned IOL and a good iridoplasty decrease the chances of the graft slipping into the vitreous cavity during surgery. However, this possibility should be kept in mind, and care should be taken to avoid any inappropriate fluidics that may cause a graft drop.

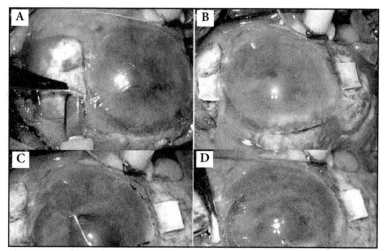

Figure 4-6. DSEK with glued IOL (part 1). (A) 2 partial thickness limbal-based scleral flaps of 2.5 × 2.5 mm are created 180 degrees opposite each other followed by placement of infusion cannula. (B) After both flaps are made, the cornea is marked with a marking pen at the center of the corneal dome, and an 8.5-mm blunt trephine is used to mark the area concentric to this mark to facilitate in Descemet's scoring and stripping. (C) After Descemet's scoring, the Descemet's membrane is stripped with a reverse Sinskey hook. (D) The IOL is held with McPherson forceps and inserted through the scleral incision. The leading haptic is grasped with microcapsulorrhexis forceps. (Reprinted with permission from Agarwal A. Femtosecond-assisted Descemet stripping automated endothelial keratoplasty with fibrin glue-assisted sutureless posterior chamber lens implantation. *Cornea.* 2010;29[11]:1315-1319.)

GLUED IOL WITH
DESCEMET'S STRIPPING
ENDOTHELIAL KERATOPLASTY

Descemet's stripping endothelial keratoplasty (DSEK) can be combined effectively with glued IOL (Figures 4-6 through 4-8). DSEK is a partial-thickness corneal graft operation in which the inner endothelial layer is replaced. The glued IOL is put in place and followed by iridoplasty, host descemetorhexis, and insertion and flotation of the DSEK graft. DSEK may cause more induced hyperopia than DMEK and PDEK, but may be preferred in cases with an incomplete iris-IOL diaphragm, large-sector iridectomies, or traumatic/congenital aniridia. The standard DSAEK graft or the ultra-thin DSEK graft may be used. The DSEK graft may be inserted using the

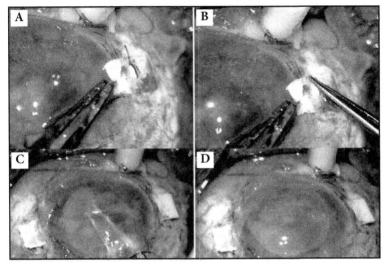

Figure 4-7. DSEK with glued IOL (part 2). (A) The trailing haptic is exteriorized via the sclerotomy. (B) The trailing haptic is tucked into the intrascleral lamellar pocket. (C) The donor lenticule is inserted into the eye. (D) The donor lenticule is unfolded with saline injection and adjusted. (Reprinted with permission from Agarwal A. Femtosecond-assisted Descemet stripping automated endothelial keratoplasty with fibrin glue-assisted sutureless posterior chamber lens implantation. *Cornea.* 2010;29[11]:1315-1319.)

taco technique with forceps, a Busin glide, a Tan endo-inserter, or the suture pull-through technique.

Two partial-thickness scleral flaps approximately 2.5 × 2.5 mm are made 180 degrees opposite each other. An AC maintainer is introduced in the inferior quadrant (Figure 4-6A). A circular mark is placed on the patient's corneal surface and serves as a guide for removal of the recipient Descemet's membrane (Figure 4-6B). The AC is entered through a peripheral stab incision, and Descemet's membrane is scored and detached as a single disc (Figure 4-6C). It is important not to damage the inner surface of the patient's cornea while removing the Descemet's membrane because the inner corneal stroma will form half of the donor/recipient interface. A sclerotomy wound is created with a 20-gauge needle approximately 1 mm away from limbus beneath the scleral flaps, and the entire glued IOL surgery is performed until the tucking of the haptics in the scleral pockets (Figure 4-6D, and Figure 4-7A and B). An inferior peripheral iridectomy is performed to prevent a postoperative air bubble-associated pupillary block glaucoma attack. An AC maintainer helps to maintain the AC throughout the surgery. The use of viscoelastic is discouraged because it is important

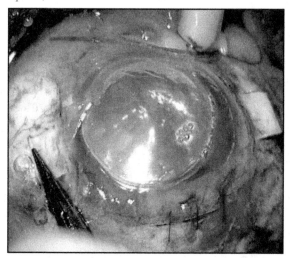

Figure 4-8. DSEK with glued IOL (part 3). Air is injected into the AC to fix the donor lenticule. Fibrin glue is used to seal the scleral flaps. (Reprinted with permission from Agarwal A. Femtosecond-assisted Descemet stripping automated endothelial keratoplasty with fibrin glue-assisted sutureless posterior chamber lens implantation. *Cornea.* 2010;29[11]:1315-1319.)

not to leave residual viscoelastic in the AC; it may potentially hamper good adhesion between the donor corneal disc and the recipient corneal stroma.

Next, the donor cornea is mounted within an artificial AC and pressurized. Manual dissection is used to remove the anterior corneal stroma. The dissected donor corneal tissue is then placed with the epithelial side down, and trephination is carried out from the endothelial side using a disposable trephine. The diameter of the trephine matches the diameter of the circular mark placed on the corneal epithelium of the recipient cornea made at the beginning of the procedure. The donor disc is about 150 microns thick.

A small amount of viscoelastic is placed on the endothelial surface of the donor corneal disc. The donor corneal disc is then introduced into the AC (Figure 4-7C) using a taco-fold technique with forceps or inserted using a surgical glide or an inserter in its unfolded or partially folded state (Figure 4-7D). Once within the AC, the donor disc is attached to the recipient's inner corneal stroma using a large air bubble (Figure 4-8). The donor/recipient interface is formed between donor and recipient corneal stroma. The donor disc is then centered on the recipient cornea using the preplaced epithelial circular mark. Approximately 10 minutes is allowed to elapse to facilitate initial donor recipient corneal disc adherence. Postoperatively, the patient is asked to lie flat in the recovery room for approximately an hour and also to lie flat for the most part during the first postoperative day.

GLUED IOL WITH DESCEMET'S MEMBRANE ENDOTHELIAL KERATOPLASTY

DMEK was described by Dr. Gerrit Melles[15] and refers to transplantation of Descemet's membrane with endothelium. It has advantages over DSAEK with respect to visual quality, absence of hyperopization, and lower rates of graft rejection. The DMEK graft may be harvested directly by the operating surgeon or may be ordered from an eye bank. The submerged cornea using backgrounds away (SCUBA) technique, as described by Dr. Arthur Giebel,[16] is used to harvest the DMEK graft. It is more harvested more easily from older donor corneas due to weaker attachments between the Descemet's membrane and pre-Descemet's layer (Dua's layer) and overlying stroma. Corneas younger than 40 years are therefore generally not suitable for DMEK. The DMEK graft is more fragile than the DSAEK and PDEK grafts and is more likely to tear during graft preparation and manipulation if handled inappropriately. Therefore, extreme care should be exercised while handling it.

Glued IOL implantation and air fill check is followed by host descemetorhexis and DMEK graft implantation. Perception of light and intraocular pressure are checked and the patient maintains a supine position for 24 hours (Figure 4-9).

In patients with compromised endothelium (Figure 4-9A), it has a tremendous potential for faster recovery. The recipient corneal dissection in DMEK is similar to that of the previous 2 procedures, resulting in the exposure of the patient's uncut inner corneal stroma. An inferior peripheral iridectomy is performed, as in DSEK and DSAEK procedures. The donor Descemet's membrane is scored, partially detached under fluid, and trephined from the endothelial side. A Sinskey hook is used to lift up the edge of the cut Descemet's membrane. Once an adequate edge is lifted, non-toothed forceps are used to gently grab the Descemet's membrane at its very edge. The graft (Figure 4-9B) is separated from the underlying stroma in a capsulorrhexis-like circumferential manner. The Descemet's membrane with the healthy donor corneal endothelium is removed as a single donor disc without any donor corneal stroma. Hence, there is no need for an artificial AC or a microkeratome in the donor tissue preparation. This donor Descemet's membrane/endothelial complex is stained with a vital dye, such as Trypan blue for visualization.

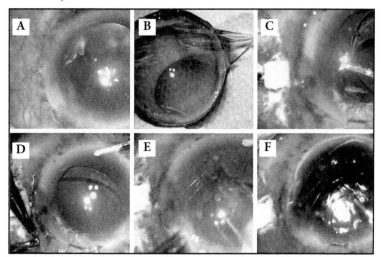

Figure 4-9. DMEK with glued IOL. (A) Preoperative pseudophakic bullous keratopathy. Note: PC IOL implanted in the AC. (B) DMEK graft being prepared. (C) PC IOL implanted in AC leading to corneal decompensation. The same PC IOL is relocated into the PC using a closed-globe glued IOL technique. The haptic is grabbed from over the iris using glued IOL forceps and the handshake technique is transferred between the 2 hands until the tip of the haptic is held. (D) The haptic is exteriorized through the sclerotomy made under the scleral flap. The same procedure is followed for the second haptic, which is exteriorized through a sclerotomy under a second scleral flap created 180 degrees from the first. Each haptic is then tucked into a scleral tunnel created at the edge of the scleral flap. (E) The DMEK graft loaded in a STAAR Implantable Collamer Lens (ICL) injector is injected into the AC. (F) The DMEK graft is unrolled, and an air bubble is used to appose it against the overlying stroma. (Reprinted with permission from Dr. Agarwal's Eye Hospital.)

An AC maintainer is introduced and all the steps of glued IOL surgery are followed consecutively, beginning from the 180-degree opposite scleral marking to the externalization and tucking of the haptics (Figure 4-9C and D). The graft is then carefully loaded into a STAAR Implantable Collamer Lens (ICL) injector (Figure 4-9E) with the cartridge tip held occluded with a finger. It is then injected gently into the AC by plunging the soft-tipped injector, taking care not to fold the graft. Wound-assisted implantation is avoided and the AC maintainer flow is titrated carefully to prevent backflow and extrusion of the graft through the incision. The default shape of the donor disc is a coiled circular tube. This donor disc is then uncoiled using fluidics, and the surgeon must avoid, for the most part, any direct instrument contact before the donor endothelium. Proper orientation is essential prior to attaching the donor Descemet's membrane to the exposed recipient bare corneal stroma. The graft orientation is then checked and it is unfolded gently using a small air bubble, as described by Melles.[15] Once unfolded, an adequately tight air bubble is injected under the graft to float it up against the stroma (Figure 4-9F). Finally, fibrin glue is used to seal the lamellar scleral flaps, conjunctiva, and clear corneal incisions.

DIFFERENCES BETWEEN DESCEMET'S STRIPPING ENDOTHELIAL KERATOPLASTY, DESCEMET'S MEMBRANE ENDOTHELIAL KERATOPLASTY, AND PRE-DESCEMET'S ENDOTHELIAL KERATOPLASTY

In DSEK, we use approximately 75 to 200 micron grafts depending on if it is ultrathin or not. Generally, with DMEK, we use 15 micron and cannot use donors aged less than 40 to 50 years. In PDEK we use 25 micron. The differences between these procedures are shown in Table 4-1.

IT TAKES TWO TO TANGO: PRE-DESCEMET'S ENDOTHELIAL KERATOPLASTY WITH GLUED IOL

PDEK was described by Agarwal and Dua.[6] Here, the newly described pre-Descemet's layer, the Descemet's membrane, and the endothelium are transplanted after host Descemet's membrane stripping. The combination of PDEK with the glued IOL procedure (Figures 4-10 through 4-12) serves to handle corneal endothelial dysfunction and secondary IOL fixation simultaneously. One important surgical step in PDEK is air pump-assisted PDEK as air is used to help unroll the PDEK graft.

Technique

A trephine of suitable diameter is used to mark the anterior corneal surface for Descemet's stripping. The desired diameter of the graft should be approximately 0.5 mm smaller than that of the recipient eye. The PDEK graft is then prepared. A 30-gauge needle attached to an air-filled 5-mL syringe is introduced in a bevel-up position into the donor corneoscleral rim placed endothelial side up. Air is then injected to form a Type 1 bubble of the

TABLE 4-1. DIFFERENCES BETWEEN DESCEMET'S STRIPPING ENDOTHELIAL KERATOPLASTY, DESCEMET'S MEMBRANE ENDOTHELIAL KERATOPLASTY, AND PRE-DESCEMET'S ENDOTHELIAL KERATOPLASTY

	DSEK	DMEK	PDEK
Technical difficulty	Easy	Difficult	Moderate
Type of procedure	Tissue additive	Tissue neutral	Minimal tissue additive
Artificial AC	Required	N/A	N/A
Microkeratome	Required (DSAEK)	N/A	N/A
Induced hyperopia	Yes	No	No
Corneal thickness	Increased	Normal	Minimal
Intrastromal interface	Yes	No	Minimal
Cost	Costly	Cost-effective	Cost-effective
Eye bank-prepared donor tissue	Available	Available	Available
Graft unrolling	Easy	Difficult	Moderate
Tissue handling	Good	Difficult	Good
Visual recovery	Slow	Fast	Good
Surgical layers	Stroma + DM + Endo	DM + Endo	Pre-Descemet's + DM + Endo

DM = Descemet's membrane; Endo = Endothelium; N/A = Not applicable

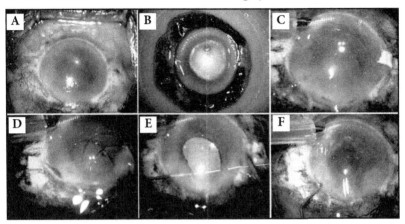

Figure 4-10. PDEK with glued IOL (part 1). (A) Preoperative photograph of the cornea of a patient with pseudophakic bullous keratopathy. PC IOL in AC. (B) A Type 1 big bubble between the pre-Descemet's layer (Dua's layer) and stroma is formed. Note the big bubble does not reach the periphery of the cornea because there are firm adhesions between the pre-Descemet's layer and stroma in the periphery. If a bubble is created that extends to the corneoscleral limbus, it is a Type 2 (pre-Descemet's) big bubble. This means the air has formed between the Descemet's membrane and the pre-Descemet's layer. (C) AC maintainer is fixed and scleral flaps are created. (D) Glued IOL surgery is performed and haptics are externalized. The same PC IOL in the AC is converted to a PC IOL in the PC with the handshake technique and glued IOL. (E) Pupilloplasty. (F) Pupilloplasty completed with glued IOL in place. Eye is now ready for PDEK surgery. (Reprinted with permission from Dr. Agarwal's Eye Hospital.)

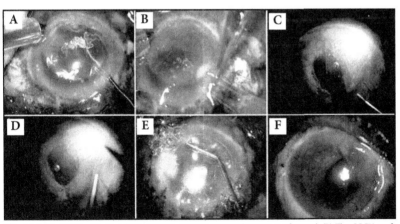

Figure 4-11. PDEK with glued IOL (part 2). (A) Descemetorhexis is performed. (B) The PDEK graft is injected into the AC with the help of the injector. (C) Graft is subsequently unrolled with air and fluidics. An endoilluminator is used to help ascertain orientation and check the unrolling of the graft. (D) The graft is unrolled after checking correct orientation. (E) Air is injected under the graft to appose it to the cornea. PDEK graft is attached to the cornea with a complete air fill of the AC, and then glue is applied to the scleral flaps. (F) One week after surgery. (Reprinted with permission from Dr. Agarwal's Eye Hospital.)

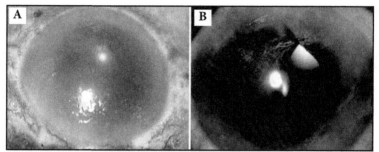

Figure 4-12. PDEK with glued IOL (part 3). (A) Preoperative case of pseudophakic bullous keratopathy with a PC IOL placed in the AC. (B) One year after surgery. (Reprinted with permission from Dr. Agarwal's Eye Hospital.)

desired diameter. The Type 1 bubble consists of the pre-Descemet's layer, the Descemet's membrane, and the endothelium and is seen as a dome-shaped elevation that is approximately 7 to 8 mm in diameter. It typically enlarges from center to the periphery and has a distinct edge all around. Trypan blue is then used to stain the graft with a 26-gauge needle introduced into the edge of the bubble once the bubble is entered with a knife. Vannas scissors are used to cut the graft all around the edges of the bubble, and the graft is harvested. It is placed into a bowl containing the storage medium. If a Type 2 bubble consisting of only Descemet's membrane and endothelium is formed, surgery may be continued as a DMEK. The Type 2 bubble is larger and enlarges from the periphery to the center. It does not have a clearly defined edge and is more likely than a Type 1 bubble to burst; therefore, care should be taken while expanding it.

The recipient eye is prepared as mentioned previously by stripping the Descemet's membrane. When combining with glued IOL surgery, the IOL implantation is completed, followed by iridoplasty and PDEK graft implantation. The graft is loaded into an IOL injector as described by Dr. Francis Price,[17] and injected into the AC. Graft orientation is confirmed, followed by unfolding and floating up of the graft using an air bubble.

The PDEK graft has advantages over the DMEK graft in that it is more robust and less likely to tear. It also allows the use of young donor grafts of any age, thereby allowing the transfer of a greater quantity of endothelial cells. This enables the use of donor grafts that are better in quality than those for DMEK.

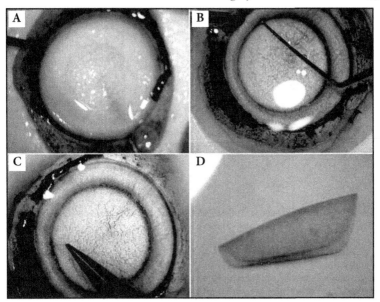

Figure 4-13. PDEK procedure converted into a DMEK procedure. A 30-gauge needle with an air-filled syringe is introduced. (A) Type 1 bubble not created. (B) A trephine marks the area of the endothelium to make the DMEK graft. (C) Donor Descemet's membrane is scored. (D) Curled DMEK graft kept in storage media. (Reprinted with permission from Dr. Agarwal's Eye Hospital.)

PRE-DESCEMET'S ENDOTHELIAL KERATOPLASTY CONVERTED TO DESCEMET'S MEMBRANE ENDOTHELIAL KERATOPLASTY

When a Type 1 bubble cannot be created, it is necessary to convert to a DMEK procedure (Figure 4-13) to avoid discarding the donor tissue. For this conversion of PDEK preparation to DMEK, an 8- to 8.5-mm trephine is used to make a mark in the endothelium. A stripper then begins to strip the endothelium from the Dua's layer. Finally, the surgeon prepares the DMEK graft.

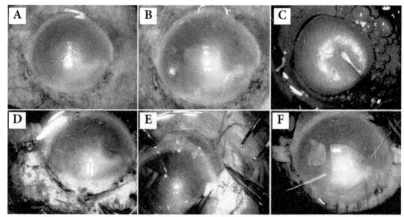

Figure 4-14. PDEK procedure with infant donor cornea (part 1). (A) Pseudophakic bullous keratopathy. Note the corneal scarring. (B) Epithelium removed. Note the subluxated IOL. (C) A 30-gauge needle attached to a 5-mL air-filled syringe is introduced in a bevel-up position from the corneoscleral rim with the endothelial side up. Air is injected, and a Type 1 bubble is formed. The donor was 9 months old. (D) IOL explanted. (E) Glued IOL implanted. (F) Pupilloplasty. (Reprinted with permission from Dr. Agarwal's Eye Hospital.)

INFANT DONORS FOR PRE-DESCEMET'S ENDOTHELIAL KERATOPLASTY

In infant/young donor tissue, the presence of strong adhesions between the Descemet's membrane and the pre-Descemet's layer obviates any chances of accidental creation of a Type 2 bubble (Figures 4-14 through 4-16). Infant donor tissue is not ideal for a DMEK procedure because it is difficult to peel the Descemet's membrane layer off the residual cornea. These adhesions help in PDEK surgery because they decrease the chances of creating a Type 2 bubble and its subsequent conversion to DMEK.

The use of infant donor cornea has an inherent advantage of abundant endothelial cells that should theoretically translate into faster resolution of corneal edema and greater longevity of grafts. The maximum endothelial cell loss in our cases occurred during the first postoperative month and it appeared to be stabilized by 6 months in all the cases. This endothelial cell loss can be attributed to either intraoperative tissue manipulation or to subsequent postoperative endothelial cell loss. The use of infant donor tissue can partly compensate for the endothelial cell loss during PDEK and keep the postoperative endothelial cell density at a high level.

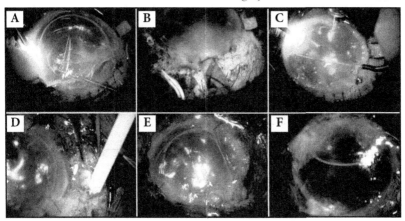

Figure 4-15. PDEK procedure with infant donor cornea (part 2). (A) Descemetorhexis is performed under air. Endoilluminator helps to enhance the visualization. (B) The infant donor graft is loaded onto the cartridge of a foldable IOL injector (the spring was removed to prevent any damage to the graft) and is slowly injected into the eye. (C) The donor graft is unrolled, and the endoilluminator helps to identify the correct graft orientation. (D) Fibrin glue is applied beneath the scleral flaps (for case 3). (E) Corneal incisions are closed with 10-0 nylon sutures, and the AC is filled with air. (F) Four days after surgery. (Reprinted with permission from Dr. Agarwal's Eye Hospital.)

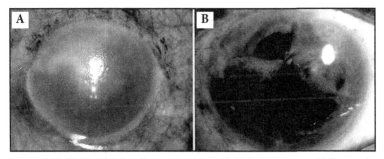

Figure 4-16. PDEK with infant donor cornea (part 3). (A) Before surgery. (B) Six months after PDEK with glued IOL. The donor was 9 months old. (Reprinted with permission from Dr. Agarwal's Eye Hospital.)

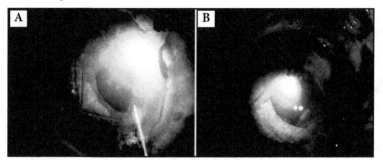

Figure 4-17. Endoilluminator-assisted PDEK. (A) PDEK graft is upside down. (B) PDEK graft on correct side. Through the endoilluminator, the rolled-up edges can be seen. (Reprinted with permission from Dr. Agarwal's Eye Hospital.)

Endoilluminator-Assisted Descemet's Membrane Endothelial Keratoplasty/Pre-Descemet's Endothelial Keratoplasty

Endoilluminator-assisted DMEK (E-DMEK) and E-PDEK (as it is referred to when applied in a PDEK; Figure 4-17) were described by Dr. Soosan Jacob. Here, the endoilluminator is used to enhance visualization and 3-dimensional depth perception of the DMEK graft. Light from the endoilluminator is shown obliquely while the microscope light is switched off. This light bouncing off the folds and edges of the DMEK graft allows very good 3-dimensional perception even in a hazy, edematous cornea. This helps the surgeon to comprehend more easily the graft position, orientation, morphology, and dynamics, all of which leads to easier and faster surgery. It avoids unnecessary maneuvers that might otherwise be required to analyze graft position and thereby decreases potential graft damage. It makes determining graft orientation with respect to endothelial vs Descemetic side a non-touch technique.

Boston Kpro With Glued IOL

A keratoprosthetic device is intended to provide a transparent optical pathway through an opacified cornea in an eye that is not a reasonable candidate for a corneal transplant. The Boston Kpro is a permanent keratoprosthetic device that has been proposed for those in whom attempts at corneal transplant have failed.

Keratoprosthetic devices differ in design, but basically consist of a special tube that acts as a visualization channel anchored to the front surface of the cornea. Implantation techniques differ, and success rates are variable and depend highly on the skill of the surgeon.

The device is available in 2 formats—Types I and II. The Type I Boston Kpro is available in either a single standard pseudophakic plano power or customized aphakic powers (based on axial length) with back plates in adult (8.5-mm diameter) and pediatric (7.0-mm diameter) sizes. The Type II format is similar, but is reserved for severe end-stage ocular surface disease desiccation that requires a permanent tarsorrhaphy to be performed, through which a small anterior nub of the Type II model protrudes.

The primary keratoprosthesis surgery is often combined with other procedures, including iridoplasty, glaucoma filtration devices, IOL and lens capsule removal, and core vitrectomy. The Boston Kpro comes with its own set of indications regarding where it can be applied and, when coupled with glued IOL, the indications become more constrained. A combined procedure can be considered for any condition associated with secondary IOL implantation for which the Boston Kpro is the only indication. The Boston Kpro comes in aphakic and pseudophakic models. If the surgeon is using a pseudophakic model and the eye is aphakic, the eye may be fixed with a glued IOL.

CONCLUSION

The glued IOL procedure can be combined with DSAEK, DMEK, and PDEK in a safe and effective manner. An iridoplasty should be done when required. In complete aniridia, it may be required to be combined with an aniridia IOL or an artificial iris.

REFERENCES

1. Agarwal A, Kumar DA, Jacob S, Baid C, Agarwal A, Srinivasan S. Fibrin glue-assisted sutureless posterior chamber intraocular lens implantation in eyes with deficient posterior capsules. *J Cataract Refract Surg.* 2008;34(9):1433-1438.
2. Prakash G, Jacob S, Kumar DA, Narsimhan S, Agarwal A, Agarwal A. Femtosecond-assisted keratoplasty with fibrin glue assisted sutureless posterior chamber lens implantation: new triple procedure. *J Cataract Refract Surg.* 2009;35(6):973-979.
3. Prakash G, Agarwal A, Jacob S, Kumar DA, Chaudhary P, Agarwal A. Femtosecond-assisted Descemet stripping automated endothelial keratoplasty with fibrin glue-assisted sutureless posterior chamber lens implantation. *Cornea.* 2010;29(11):1315-1319.

4. Jacob S, Agarwal A, Kumar D, Agarwal A, Agarwal A, Satish K. Modified technique for combining DMEK with glued intrascleral haptic fixation of a posterior chamber IOL as a single-stage procedure. *J Refract Surg.* 2014;30(7):492-496.

5. McKee Y, Price FW Jr, Feng MT, Price MO. Implementation of the posterior chamber intraocular lens intrascleral haptic fixation technique (glued intraocular lens) in a United States practice: outcomes and insights. *J Cataract Refract Surg.* 2014;40(12):2099-2105.

6. Agarwal A, Dua HS, Narang P, et al. Pre-Descemet's endothelial keratoplasty (PDEK). *Br J Ophthalmol.* 2014;98(9):1181-1185.

7. Osher RH, Snyder ME, Cionni RJ. Modification of the Siepser slipknot technique. *J Cataract Refract Surg.* 2005;31(6):1098-1100.

8. Dua HS, Faraj LA, Said DG, et al. A novel pre-Descemet's layer (Dua's layer). *Ophthalmology.* 2013;120(9):1778-1785.

9. Agarwal A, Jacob S, Kumar DA, Agarwal A, Narsimhan S, Agarwal A. Handshake technique for glued intrascleral fixation of a posterior chamber intraocular lens. *J Cataract Refract Surg.* 2013;39(3):317-322.

10. Gabor SGB, Pavilidis MM. Sutureless intrascleral posterior chamber intraocular lens fixation. *J Cataract Refract Surg.* 2007;33(11):1851-1854.

11. Price FW Jr, Price MO. Descemet's stripping with endothelial keratoplasty in 200 eyes: early challenges and technique to enhance donor adherence. *J Cataract Refract Surg.* 2006;32(3):411-418.

12. Jacob S, Agarwal A, Agarwal A, Narasimhan S, Kumar DA, Sivagnanam S. Endo illuminator-assisted transcorneal illumination for Descemet's membrane endothelial keratoplasty: enhanced intraoperative visualization of the graft in corneal decompensation secondary to pseudophakic bullous keratopathy. *J Cataract Refract Surg.* 2014;40(8):1332-1336.

13. Schoenberg ED, Price FW Jr. Modification of Siepser sliding suture technique for iris repair and endothelial keratoplasty. *J Cataract Refract Surg.* 2014;40(5):705-708.

14. Prakash G, Jacob S, Kumar AD, Narsimhan S, Agarwal A, Agarwal A. Femtosecond-assisted keratoplasty with fibrin glue-assisted sutureless posterior chamber lens implantation: new triple procedure. *J Cataract Refract Surg.* 2009;35(6):973-979.

15. Dapena I, Ham L, Melles GR. Endothelial keratoplasty: DSEK/DSAEK or DMEK— the thinner the better? *Curr Opin Ophthalmol.* 2009;20(4):299-307.

16. Guerra FP, Anshu A, Price MO, Giebel AW, Price FW. Descemet's membrane endothelial keratoplasty: prospective study of 1-year visual outcomes, graft survival, and endothelial cell loss. *Ophthalmology.* 2011;118(12):2368-2373.

17. Price FW Jr, Feng MT, Price MO. Evolution of endothelial keratoplasty: where are we headed? *Cornea.* 2015 Oct;34(Suppl10):S41-S47.

5

Results and Complications of Glued IOL Surgery

Dhivya Ashok Kumar, MD *and Amar Agarwal, MS, FRCS, FRCOphth*

Glued IOL surgery involves the transscleral fixation of a posterior chamber (PC) intraocular lens (IOL) with fibrin or tissue glue in eyes with inadequate capsular support. As the name indicates, the IOL is "glued" to the eye and not sutured. Since its introduction, this technique has evolved and extended its application with excellent results.[1-38] Intraoperative capsular loss, zonular dialysis, congenital subluxated lens, ectopia lentis, and traumatic subluxation are the common surgical indications. There is no doubt that the extraordinary results in aphakic eyes with improvement in quality of vision has left patients spectacle free for distant vision after glued IOL.[1-21] Glued IOL involves modification of the Scharioth tunnel technique in which scleral flaps are used to close the haptics.[22] The glued IOL technique differs from other sutureless methods because fibrin glue is used, which enhances the rate of adhesion with hemostasis, and also because available IOLs can be used, unlike other techniques that require newly designed IOLs.[22,23] The additional advantages of this technique are the speed and ease of performance; as the time taken in suture scleral fixated IOL for passing suture is significantly reduced. The frequent complications of secondary IOL

Agarwal A, ed.
A Video Textbook of Glued IOLs (pp 99-121).
© 2016 Taylor & Francis Group.

implantation, such as secondary glaucoma, cystoid macular edema, uveitis, glaucoma, and hyphema syndrome or bullous keratopathy, are reduced.[9,11,12,16] Suture-related complications of scleral fixated IOLs, such as suture erosion, knot exposure or dislocation of the IOL after suture disintegration, or broken sutures are prevented. Although it is free from conventional suture-related complications of sutured scleral fixated IOL, a glued IOL can result in complications intraoperatively and postoperatively if not managed well. Although the surgeon's skill is one of the key factors in handling these complicated eyes, patient selection, type of IOL, preoperative workup, and postoperative follow-up are crucial for minimizing and managing complications. In this chapter, we share the results, complications, and special indications for glued IOL surgery.

VISUAL OUTCOMES AND RESULTS OF GLUED IOL SURGERY

Since the introduction of glued IOLs for deficient capsular support, the postoperative outcomes and surgical results in the short, interim, and long term have been satisfactory.[1-21,24-26] In this section, we discuss the results reported in the literature on the glued IOL procedure. In a 1-year follow-up study of 53 eyes, there was significant improvement in uncorrected visual acuity (UCVA) and spectacle best-corrected visual acuity (BCVA).[3] In our earlier report on the interim results of rigid glued IOLs (n = 152), there were significant improvements in UCVA and BCVA; 52% gained 20/20 BCVA postoperatively.[4] In a pediatric eye study, the mean postoperative BCVA was 0.43 ± 0.33, and there was a significant change noted (p < .001).[6] Postoperatively, 20/20 and greater than 20/60 BCVAs were obtained in 17.1% and 46.3% of eyes, respectively.[6] BCVA improvement of more than one line was seen in 53.6% of eyes. Prakash et al reported 3 eyes in which the same PC IOL was translocated from the anterior chamber (AC) to the PC without complications.[7] Sinha et al reported outcomes after repositioning a decentered PC IOL in the PC using the same IOL with the glued IOL method and showed good results.[11] In a comparative study by Ganekal et al, BCVA of 20/40 or better was obtained in 88% and 84% after sutured scleral fixated and glued IOL eyes, respectively.[12] In another retrospective analysis of visual outcomes that included 735 eyes, there were 486 rigid glued IOLs, 191 foldable IOLs, 10 glued iris prostheses, 16 glued IOLs with pupilloplasty, and 32 glued IOLs with penetrating keratoplasty.[9] The mean postoperative UCVA and BCVA were 0.19 ± 0.19 and 0.38 ± 0.27, respectively, in rigid IOLs (single-piece polymethylmethacrylate [PMMA] IOLs [Appasamy

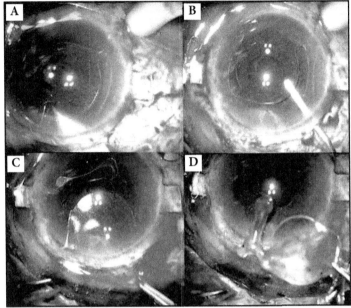

Figure 5-1. Anterior chamber IOL explanted in an eye with chronic AC IOL-induced uveitis. (A,B) Diagonal scleral flaps and superior corneo-limbal incision made. (C,D) AC IOL explanted.

Associates]). The most common indication was posterior capsular rupture (PCR) and aphakia in that report of 735 eyes. There were significant improvements in UCVA and BCVA (paired t-test, P = 0.000).[9] An additional interim study on rigid glued IOLs (PMMA) (n = 152), with a mean follow-up time of 9.7 ± 3.2 months, approximately 38.8% eyes completed > 12 months of follow-up also showed satisfactory outcomes.[4] Of 152 eyes, 116 (76.3%) and 36 (23.68%) eyes out of 152 eyes underwent the surgery as a primary or secondary procedure, respectively. The most common indication was PCR with no sulcus support (56%), followed by subluxated cataract (21%). Eight of 152 eyes underwent IOL exchange, of which 6 eyes had AC IOL (Figure 5-1) and 2 eyes had sutured scleral fixated IOL. The most common indication for IOL exchange was uveitis, and significant improvement was noted in the postoperative period according to a subjective questionnaire. A single-piece PMMA IOL with an optic size of 6.5 mm and overall diameter of 13 mm was implanted in each of those eyes.[4] The mean preoperative UCVA in decimal equivalents was 0.024 ± 0.02 and the mean postoperative UCVA at the last follow-up was 0.53 ± 0.26. There was significant improvement in UCVA. The mean preoperative and postoperative BCVAs were

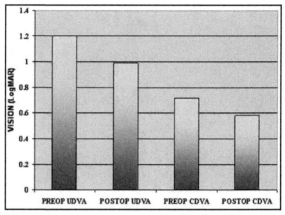

Figure 5-2. Visual outcome in foldable glued IOL. CDVA, logMAR, UDVA. (Reprinted with permission from Agarwal, A. Complications and visual outcomes after glued foldable intraocular lens implantation in eyes with inadequate capsules. *J Cataract Refract Surg.* 2013;39[8]:1211-1218.)

0.71 ± 0.26 and 0.80 ± 0.21, respectively. Of 152 eyes, 79 (52%) gained 20/20 visual acuity by 1 month after surgery.[4]

In a recent study of glued IOLs in the United States, McKee et al[27] showed mean visual acuity improvement from 20/200 to 20/50 postoperatively. Narang and Narang[28] showed that approximately 84% of eyes gained one or more lines after glued IOL surgery in eyes with inadequate capsules. Postoperatively, there was a significant improvement in the UCVA ($P < .05$) and the BCVA ($P < .05$).[28] Even in multifocal IOLs, glued IOLs have shown promising results.[4] The mean preoperative BCVA was 0.60 ± 0.25 and the mean postoperative BCVA was 0.7 ± 0.34. The postoperative mean additional add for best near corrected vision was 0.5 ± 1.1 diopters (D). There was a significant decrease in the near addition ($P = .000$). Good patient satisfaction was achieved. Serial digital slit lamp images of the eye with full pupillary dilation showed good IOL centration.[4]

In our recent series of foldable glued IOLs (n = 208), the mean uncorrected distance visual acuity (UDVA) was 1.20 ± 0.5 logMAR preoperatively and 0.99 ± 0.5 logMAR postoperatively (Figure 5-2).[24] There were significant improvements in UDVA ($P < .05$, Wilcoxon signed-rank test) and corrected distance visual acuity (CDVA) ($P < .05$) in the operated eyes. One hundred thirty (62.5%) eyes showed improvement from the preoperative CDVA. The postoperative CDVA were 20/40 or better and 20/60 or better in 81 (38.9%) and 101 (48.5%) eyes, respectively. Overall, 176 eyes (84.6%) achieved a final CDVA better than or the same as that recorded preoperatively. In

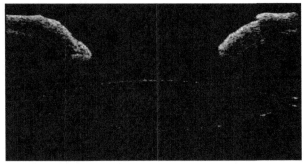

Figure 5-3. Glued IOL position as seen in optical coherence tomography.

another review of foldable glued IOLs (n = 191), with a mean follow-up of 16.6 ± 8.8 months (range: 6 to 48 months), the mean postoperative BCVA and UCVA were 0.39 ± 0.29 and 0.22 ± 0.23, respectively.[9]

In the long-term follow-up study, the mean postoperative BCVA was 0.63 ± 0.2 decimal equivalent.[15] After eliminating the eyes with comorbidity, the BCVAs of 46 eyes correlated with ocular residual astigmatism (ORA). There was a weak correlation (P = 0.013; r = −0.363) between the ORA and the BCVA. The overall mean corneal astigmatism was 1.48 ± 1.1 D. Corneal astigmatism was noted to be higher (P = 0.007) in the rigid IOL group (1.7 ± 1 D) compared with the foldable IOL group (0.98 ± 1.2), and there was no correlation (P = 0.080; r = −0.228) noted between the corneal astigmatism and visual acuity.[15] In an IOL tilt analysis study by optical coherence tomography (OCT), out of 60 eyes, optic tilt was detected in 21 (35%); no optic tilt was detected with optical coherence tomography (OCT) in 39 eyes (65%).[15] The mean angle between the IOL and the iris was noted to be 3.2 ± 2.7 degrees on the horizontal axis and 2.9 ± 2.6 degrees on the vertical axis (Figure 5-3). No association was noted between the IOL tilt and BCVA ($\chi2$ test, P = .468).[15] In an ultrasound biomicroscopic analysis of IOL position, 17.4% microscopic tilt was noted at follow-up times that ranged from 6 to 56 months.[26] The mean positions of the IOL optic from the iris pigment epithelium were 0.66 ± 0.42 mm (superior), 0.68 ± 0.42 mm (inferior), 0.63 ± 0.39 mm (nasal), and 0.61 ± 0.38 mm (temporal). Of 92 haptics examined, 85 (92.4%) were in the sulcus (Figure 5-4) and 7 (7.6%) were in the ciliary process of the pars plicata (Figure 5-5). All the IOLs had the haptics oriented in the horizontal axis. Three of 7 haptics in the ciliary process had the other haptic in the sulcus and measured optic tilt (as determined with ultrasound biomicroscopic [UBM] analysis) of more than 100 mm (Figure 5-6). The mean CDVA was 0.63 ± 0.3 (Snellen decimal equivalent). The

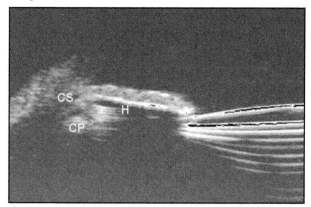

Figure 5-4. Ultrasound biomicroscopic image showing the haptic above the ciliary process in the ciliary sulcus. (Reprinted with permission from Agarwal A, Kumar DA, Packialakshmi S, Agarwal A. In vivo analysis of glued intraocular lens position with ultrasound biomicroscopy. *J Cataract Refract Surg.* 2013;39[7]:1017-1022.)

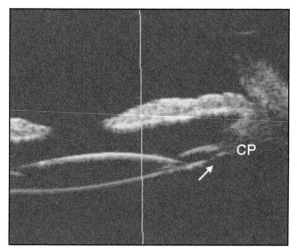

Figure 5-5. Ultrasound biomicroscopic image showing the haptic (arrow) in the ciliary process. (Reprinted with permission from Agarwal A, Kumar DA, Packialakshmi S, Agarwal A. In vivo analysis of glued intraocular lens position with ultrasound biomicroscopy. *J Cataract Refract Surg.* 2013;39[7]:1017-1022.)

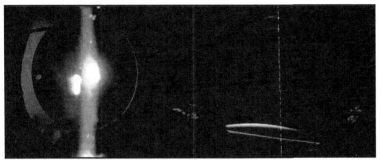

Figure 5-6. Clinical photograph (left) and UBM image (right) showing the optic tilt in an eye with one haptic in the sulcus and the other haptic in the pars plicata. (Reprinted with permission from Agarwal A, Kumar DA, Packialakshmi S, Agarwal A. In vivo analysis of glued intraocular lens position with ultrasound biomicroscopy. *J Cataract Refract Surg.* 2013;39[7]:1017-1022.)

mean postoperative refractive error was -1.2 ± 1.2 D. There was no significant difference in UDVA ($p = 0.639$) or CDVA ($p = 0.988$) between the eyes with tilt and the eyes without tilt. There was no significant difference in the postoperative cylindrical error between the eyes with tilt and the eyes without tilt ($P = .977$). There was no correlation between tilt in the vertical axis and CDVA ($P = 0.880$, Spearman correlation) or postoperative cylinder ($P = 0.841$).[26]

IOL STABILITY IN GLUED IOL SURGERY

IOL dislocation is one of the main problems associated with transscleral fixation of suture-fixated IOLs. However, in our technique, the IOL haptic is secured inside scleral pockets at the site where the tip is externalized. We routinely tuck the haptic tip inside a scleral tunnel made with a 26-gauge needle. Another concern is the change in the properties of the biomaterial when the IOL is placed in a stretched position. The 2 factors that contribute to the ability of IOL loops to maintain their original symmetrical configuration are loop rigidity (the resistance of the haptic to external forces that bend the loops centrally) and loop memory (the ability of the loops to re-expand laterally to their original size and configuration). These factors can be demonstrated by compressing or stretching the haptics in vivo (Figure 5-7). In vivo, the centrifugal force vector due to resistance to compression by the capsular bag keeps the IOL stable (Figure 5-8A). Similarly, stretch creates a centripetal resistance force, which, along with the intralamellar scleral tuck, stabilizes the IOL (Figure 5-8B). Although complete scleral wound healing with collagen fibrils may take up to 3 months, the IOL remains stable

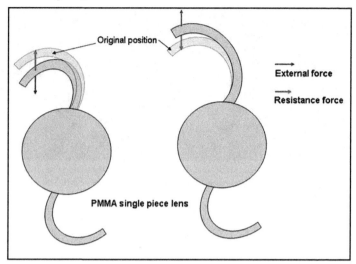

Figure 5-7. Ex vivo vector diagram showing the effect of compression and stretching on the IOL haptic. (Reprinted with permission from Agarwal A, Kumar DA, Jacob S, Prakash G. Reply: Fibrin glue-assisted sutureless scleral fixation. *J Cataract Refract Surg.* 2009;35[5]:795-796.)

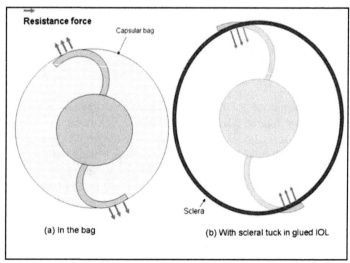

Figure 5-8. In vivo force vector diagram. (A) Centrifugal force vector due to resistance to compression by the capsular bag keeps the IOL stable. (B) In the glued IOL, the stretch creates a centripetal resistance force; along with the intralamellar scleral tuck, it stabilizes the IOL. (Reprinted with permission from Agarwal A, Kumar DA, Jacob S, Prakash G. Reply: Fibrin glue-assisted sutureless scleral fixation. *J Cataract Refract Surg.* 2009;35[5]:795-796.)

because the haptic is placed snugly inside a scleral pocket. IOL centration/ tilt was followed clinically and with anterior segment OCT. The difference between the topographic (Orbscan) and manifest refraction was constant in all eyes during the entire postoperative period, which suggests minimal new IOL-induced astigmatism. Moreover, the stability of the IOL is well maintained by the tucking procedure.

INTRAOPERATIVE COMPLICATIONS

Starting from the initial steps of creating partial-thickness scleral flaps to the final step of applying fibrin glue application, each step must be learned and achieved with perfection. Proper preoperative evaluation of intraocular pressure (IOP), scleral anomalies, and posterior segment examination are highly useful in preventing intraoperative and postoperative complications.

Nondiagonal Scleral Flaps

Scleral flaps should be 180 degrees apart diagonally. Nondiagonal flaps of 5 to 10 degrees can affect the final positioning of the IOL (Figure 5-9). Surgery should not proceed with eccentric flaps because sclerotomy must be done beneath these flaps and a path created for externalization of the haptics. This eventually leads to decentration of the IOL (Figure 5-10). A fresh flap should be created diagonally opposite to the previous one, and then the surgery can proceed.

Torn Scleral Flaps

Too much pressure on the scleral flap edges can tear the flaps and lead to loss of scleral tissue. In such a situation, new flaps should be dissected.

Small Scleral Flaps

Normal scleral flaps measure about 2.5 × 2.5 mm. Flaps smaller than 2 mm are difficult to handle and often get damaged. Flaps that are too narrow should be avoided because it may be difficult to create the scleral pocket next to the sclerotomy.

Large Scleral Flaps

When the flaps are too wide or too large, the length of the haptic underneath the flaps is longer than the one in the scleral tunnel (Figure 5-11). This problem should be avoided because longer haptic length is wasted from the

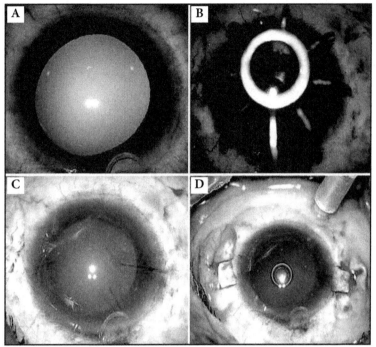

Figure 5-9. Eccentric flaps. (A) Aphakic eye for glued IOL surgery. (B) Scleral flap marker. (C) Note the sclera marking (violet mark) is eccentric. (D) Scleral flaps created are eccentric. The flaps should be 180 degrees apart. Note the flaps are about 160 degrees apart, which will lead to a decentered IOL.

sclerotomy site to the entry point of the scleral pocket. As a result, the proportion of the tucked haptic is smaller.

Disproportionate Flap Size

The amount of haptic tucked on either side is responsible for the stability of the IOL. If the amount of haptic tucked is not equal on both sides, then torsional instability can occur. Creating grafts size symmetrical on both sides is crucial for preventing this complication.

Thin Flaps

Normal scleral flap thickness should be partial or lamellar (approximately 40% depth). Superficial flaps can lead to postoperative thinning or erosion of haptics. Intraoperatively, this complication can be prevented by obtaining the exact depth of flaps and the proper dissection plane.

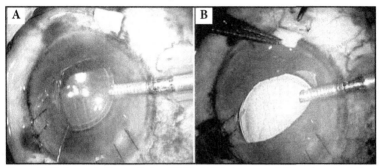

Figure 5-10. Eccentric flaps solution. (A) Glued IOL decentered. Note the scleral flaps are eccentric and not 180 degrees apart. Note the faint violet mark in the lower left corner where the flap is, but there is no marker in the upper-right corner, which led to the eccentric flap. (B) Glued IOL centered. A fresh sclerotomy is made in the upper right flap so that the 2 sclerotomies are 180 degrees apart. The IOL is again passed back into the vitreous cavity and externalized through the fresh sclerotomy. The IOL is now centered. If the flap is very badly decentered, a fresh flap would have to be made. (Reprinted with permission from Dr. Agarwal's Eye Hospital.)

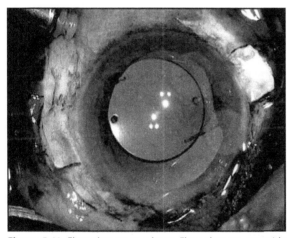

Figure 5-11. Flaps that are too large. Flaps that are too wide should be avoided because a longer haptic length is wasted from the sclerotomy site to the entry point of the scleral pocket. As a result, very little haptic is available for tucking. (Reprinted with permission from Dr. Agarwal's Eye Hospital.)

Premature Scleral Entry

Accidental scleral entry while dissecting the scleral flaps rarely occurs. This can be prevented by positioning the keratome bevel up throughout the dissection.

Anterior Sclerotomy

The sclerotomy should be placed 1.0 to 1.5 mm from the limbus. An anteriorly (< 1 mm) placed sclerotomy will lead to injury to the iris root and sometimes bleeding. Haptic externalization and tucking into the scleral tunnel will also be affected. Therefore, an anterior sclerotomy should be closed with sutures, and another sclerotomy should be made behind it to externalize the haptic.

Posterior Sclerotomy

A sclerotomy placed more than 2 mm from the limbus risks exposure to microbes because it is closer to the flap edge. Because a longer haptic length is wasted from the limbus to the sclerotomy site, there is very little haptic left behind to tuck. In this situation, the haptic should be reinternalized, a new sclerotomy should be made 1.0 mm from the limbus, and the haptic should be re-externalized.[29] If necessary, a pupilloplasty may be done to prevent optic capture.

Vitrectomy-Related Complications

During the learning curve, vitrectomy-related challenges may be encountered in the glued IOL procedure. Incomplete vitrectomy and iris damage can occur during vitreous cutting. Undue traction or excess suction can be better avoided. Triamcinolone can be used to stain the vitreous, which ensures that no vitreous strand is present in the AC and the pupil is completely free from vitreous. Vitrectomy can be done from the corneal incision (using a 20-gauge cutter) or from the sclerotomy site with a 23- or 25-gauge cutter. The vitreous is removed to a level just posterior to the capsule. Improper vitreous removal can lead to pupil peaking and late retinal traction.

Intraoperative Hyphema

Inadvertent damage to the iris or inflamed eye with previous neovascularization can lead to intraoperative hyphema. It can also be caused by a forceful, sudden entry through the iris root in an anterior sclerotomy.

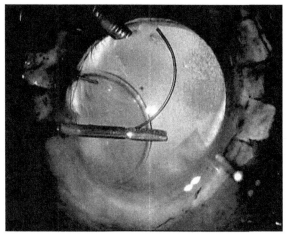

Figure 5-12. Broken IOL haptic. (Reprinted with permission from Dr. Agarwal's Eye Hospital.)

Patients with proliferative eye diseases such as diabetes or neovascular glaucoma are predisposed to intraoperative hyphema.

Iridodialysis

Forceful sclerotomy entry at the limbus can lead to detachment of the iris from its root and iridodialysis. Any resistance encountered during sclerotomy should be taken as a warning sign, and the needle should be withdrawn. Once resistance is felt at the entry site, it is better to withdraw the needle and re-enter in the adjacent site. Large iridodialyses should be sutured intraoperatively by using a modified Siepser slip knot.

Broken Haptic

Undue pressure at the haptic tip can cause haptic breakage. Kinking and bent haptic tips have also been seen in modified PMMA-type or prolene haptics. Avoiding undue pressure, following the curve of the IOL, using exact forceps for holding the tips, and mastering the handshake technique will reduce haptic-related complications. Single-piece IOLs with rigid haptics are more prone to breakage due to their rigidity and lack of tensile strength (Figures 5-12 and 5-13). Breakage can occur in the tip, away from the tip, or in the haptic optic junction. Whenever the haptic is broken, it must be replaced with another IOL. A foldable glued IOL study reported 0.4% haptic breakage (n = 1), which was immediately replaced with another IOL.[24] There was haptic deformation in 2 eyes (0.9%).[24]

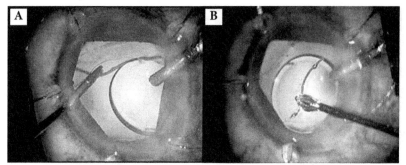

Figure 5-13. Haptic breakage. (A) IOL haptic deformed with the glued IOL forceps. (B) IOL haptic broken. (Reprinted with permission from Dr. Agarwal's Eye Hospital.)

IOL Drop

IOL drop is usually encountered in the early stages of the surgeon's learning curve. Because there is no PC available for support, any error on the part of the surgeon during the handling of the IOL can lead to an IOL drop. Sudden and uncontrolled unfolding of the IOL during injection can cause this complication; therefore, unfolding of the IOL should always be gradual and slow.[30] Inadvertent dropping or slipping of the haptic happens when the surgeon is not well trained in the handshake technique. This can also happen when the externalized haptic is not stabilized properly. Use of silicone tires to stabilize the externalized haptic was introduced by Beiko and Steinert[31] to reduce this complication. Improper handling of the haptic by a surgeon or failure of the assistant to hold the externalized haptic may cause the haptic to slip back into the eye.

Corneal Damage

An IOL injection that is wound too tightly can induce pressure on the margins and the endothelium of the cornea. It is better to avoid wound-assisted injection, and care should be taken while externalizing the trailing haptic, so that no endothelial damage is occurring. While using an AC maintainer, make sure that the tip is not damaging the corneal Descemet membrane.

Decentered IOL

The partial-thickness scleral flaps must be created exactly 180 degrees opposite each another. Eccentric flaps lead to a decentered IOL because the haptics are externalized beneath the flaps from the sclerotomy site. When

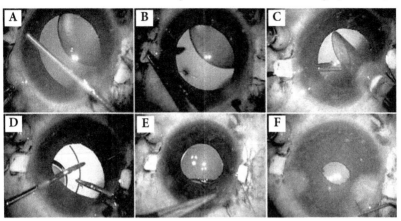

Figure 5-14. Peripheral iridectomy in large eyes. (A) Vitrector assisted peripheral iridectomy is done at the base of the scleral flap in an eye with large white-to-white (WTW) diameter. (B) Anterior sclerotomy is performed about 0.5 mm away from the limbus and the needle enters the eye without injuring the base of iris or causing any undue traction. (C) 23-gauge glued IOL forceps are introduced from the sclerotomy site and they grasp the tip of the 3-piece foldable IOL. (D) Handshake technique being done for externalization of the trailing haptic. (E) Both the haptics are externalized. (F) Wound sutured and hydration done. Note the peripheral iridectomies position and well-placed IOL.

the IOL is not positioned along its long axis, continuous stress on the haptics leads to decentration. In such cases, fresh flaps should be created exactly opposite each other, and externalization of the haptic should be redone on one side.[30] Improper or asymmetrical haptics lead to decentration. Decentered IOLs can be seen intraoperatively by determining the optic in relation to the pupil (if it is round) or with respect to the limbus diameter.

Lack of Haptic Length

Eyes with a large white-to-white diameter and the conventional or horizontal scleral flaps at 3 o'clock and 9 o'clock may cause lack of or inadequate haptic for tucking. A vertical glued IOL procedure can be performed in these cases, with the flaps oriented at 12 o'clock and 6 o'clock, respectively. The vertical white-to-white (WTW) diameter is less than that of the horizontal WTW diameter. Keratoglobus, high myopia, and megalocornea are some of the conditions where the corneal diameter may be high. In large eyes, peripheral iridectomy can be electively made exactly at the base of the scleral flaps (Figure 5-14). This will prevent undue traction on the iris and gives room for the IOL haptic to be mobilized with ease. This simple method helps to avoid any iatrogenic iris tissue damage during the surgical procedure.

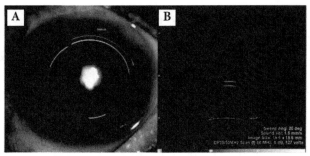

Figure 5-15. (A) Postoperative glued IOL. (B) Ultrasound microscopic image of the IOL without tilt.

Imbrication of IOL

In large eyes, the haptic is imbricated to the sclera with 10-0 prolene suture for better stabilization. This has been introduced by Dr. Sadeer Hanush and Dr. Yuri Mckee.

Tilted IOL

A tilted IOL can occur if the IOL is not centered well. Any difference in the positions of the 2 sclerotomy ports can affect the final position of the haptic and can induce optic tilt. This complication was shown in our study, in which 3 of 8 eyes with one haptic in the ciliary sulcus and the other in the pars plicata had a tilt of more than 100 mm.[26] Two eyes had both haptics in the pars plicata but with no optic tilt. Because the positions of externalization were equal on both sides, no significant tilt was observed on UBM (Figure 5-15). Incarcerating a longer part of the haptic stabilizes the axial position of the PC IOL, leading to a decrease in the incidence of IOL tilt. However, in our series, there was no association between optic tilt and haptic location ($P = .585$, χ^2 test). As with any surgical technique, the surgeon aims for equidistant placement of the haptics; however, in some cases, the desired configuration cannot be attained with absolute certainty. Anatomic or structural features, such as capsule remnants, vitreous, coagulated blood, or small membranes, may interfere with the optimum positions of the haptics.

Correct Shake for Handshake

The operating surgeon sometimes struggles during haptic externalization due to an incorrect sitting position in relation to the plane of scleral

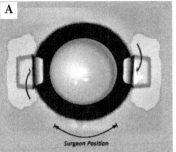

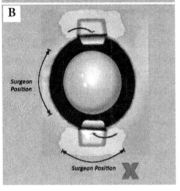

Figure 5-16. (A) The scleral flaps are positioned horizontally and the surgeon sits almost perpendicular to the plane of haptic manipulation. (B) This image demonstrates the scleral flaps that are made at 12 and 6 'o clock positions. If the surgeon positions at the same plane as that of the plane of haptic externalization for handshake, difficulty in manipulation is encountered. When the surgeon shifts temporally, the position is apt and the haptics can be easily manipulated with the correct shake for handshake technique.

flaps and the plane of haptic manipulation. Positioning the surgeon is crucial for performing the correct handshake technique without difficulty (Figure 5-16) and thereby externalizing the haptics. The plane of scleral flaps and the plane of performing a handshake should be perpendicular to the surgeon's position (ie, when horizontal flaps are made at 3 o'clock and 9 o'clock hours, the surgeon should sit superior at 12 o'clock, and when vertical flaps are made at 12 o'clock and 6 o'clock hours, the surgeon should sit temporally.

POSTOPERATIVE COMPLICATIONS

Corneal Edema

Excessive intraoperative damage to the endothelial cells or cornea can lead to immediate postoperative corneal edema. It usually resolves within 2 to 3 days with medical management. This complication may occur in the early learning curve of the technique, and once the surgical skills are mastered, it can be overcome.

Intraocular Lens Tilt

The accurate position of an IOL in the capsular bag is vital for preventing postoperative tilt and astigmatism. IOL tilt is one of the components of malposition that can lead to astigmatism, change in optical higher-order aberrations, and loss of BCVA. Symmetrical positioning of the sclerotomies is one of the key steps in achieving a stable glued IOL. Any difference in the 2 sclerotomy wounds can affect the final position of the haptic and can induce optic tilt. Incarcerating a longer part of the haptic stabilizes the axial position of the PC IOL, leading to a decrease in the incidence of IOL tilt (see Figure 5-14). A UBM analysis of postoperative glued IOLs found microscopic tilt in 17.4% of the eyes.[26] Eight (17.4%) of 46 eyes had optic tilt of more than 100 mm; the difference was in the vertical axis (superior–inferior) in 7 (15.2%) eyes and in the horizontal axis (nasal–temporal) in 1 (2.1%) eye. In the eyes with tilt, there were 4 foldable IOLs and 4 rigid IOLs. The difference in the optic position between the eyes with tilt and eyes without tilt was more in the nasal position. There was no significant association between the presence of optic tilt and haptic location ($P = .585$, χ2 test). There was no significant difference ($P = .077$) in the ORA between eyes with optic tilt and eyes without optic tilt on UBM. The optic tilt noted in our study was less than the tilt seen in scleral fixated IOLs, as reported by Loya et al[32] and Swelam et al.[33] Asymmetric attachment of the sutures to the haptics, failure to place the needles through the sclera 180 degrees apart, and suture loosening, breakage, or slippage on the haptics can also result in IOL tilt with suture-fixated PC IOLs. However, with the glued IOL technique, there is no anchoring of haptics with sutures; hence, there are no suture or haptic problems.

In our long-term IOL tilt analysis by OCT, we noted that of 60 eyes, optic tilt was detected in 21 (35%); in 39 eyes (65%), no optic tilt was detected on OCT. The mean angles between the IOL and the iris were noted to be 3.2 ± 2.7 on the horizontal axis and 2.9 ± 2.6 on the vertical axis. No association was noted between IOL tilt and BCVA ($P = .468$, χ2 test). In our series, the IOL tilt was noted to induce no significant astigmatism in the operated eyes in the long term.[15]

Early IOL Decentration

Asymmetric scleral flaps, nondiagonal flaps, and unequal haptic tucking are the common causes of early postoperative IOL decentration. Immediate

IOL repositioning in the operating room is advised in such situations. In our foldable glued IOL series, IOL decentration was seen in 3.3% of the cases.[24] During repositioning, it was noted that improper intrascleral haptic tuck was the reason for IOL decentration. Late IOL decentration was less frequent in the foldable glued IOL study than in our previous study of rigid IOLs. Unequal haptic tuck on both scleral tunnels will lead to late IOL decentration. Undue pressure on the haptic tip can cause haptic deformation and later dislodgement. However, in our series, eyes with intraoperative haptic deformation did not have late decentration. The overall diameter of the IOL can also affect the centration of the IOL. An especially large diameter can provide better IOL centration; however, in our series, we did not use large-diameter IOLs.

Late IOL Decentration

Late IOL decentration is rare with the glued IOL procedure. Once the IOL is noted to be stable postoperatively, the risk of decentration is lower. A 1-year study of IOL decentration or shift showed that the mean x- and y-axis shift was 0.091 ± 0.19 mm and 0.019 ± 0.05 mm, respectively.[3] There was no significant change in x-axis shift in the postoperative follow-up period (Wilcoxon signed-rank test, $P = 1.00$).

Haptic Extrusion

Improper haptic tuck and scleral flaps that are too thin can lead to haptic extrusion. In this situation, the haptic must be retucked into the correct scleral tunnel. Proper conjunctival apposition is also important for providing additional adhesive effect on the sclera.

Subconjunctival Haptic

Proper scleral closure and conjunctival apposition is crucial for preventing subconjunctival haptic erosion. Eyes with flaps that are too thin, excessive use of scleral cautery, and scleral thinning disorders, such as rheumatoid arthritis, are more prone to such a complication. If the haptic is below the conjunctiva, the IOL is well centered, and the patient does not have any complaints, there is no need for surgical intervention. However, if it is exposed, it must be refixed.

Glaucoma

Postoperative glaucoma was not reported in our 1-year follow-up of glued IOL or in our pediatric glued IOL case series. However, there was one (0.4%)

eye that had ocular hypertension (>21 mm Hg) postoperatively and was treated medically.[24] The risk of glaucoma with this technique is expected to be lower, unlike with AC or sutured scleral fixated IOLs, because there is no angle damage or chronic iris chafing. Patients at high risk for postoperative secondary glaucoma include those with previous uveitis, trauma, and steroid response. Therefore, IOP needs to be continuously monitored in all patients who have undergone glued IOL surgery.

Cystoid Macular Edema

Complicated cataract surgery and prolonged surgical manipulation with vitreous loss can predispose patients to cystoid macular edema (CME). The loss of CDVA postoperatively occurred due to CME in 4 (1.9%) of eyes with a foldable glued IOL.[24] In the pediatric age group, the incidence of postoperative macular edema was 4.8% (n = 2).[6] Another report showed 7.5% healed macular changes after glued IOL surgery by the 1-year follow-up.[3]

Retinal Detachment

Vitrectomy at the sclerotomy site is crucial for preventing postoperative retinal traction. Inadequate or improper vitrectomy across the pupillary plane and sclerotomy port leads to postoperative retinal traction and breaks. Eyes with trauma, a dislocated IOL, or previous retinal traction are at risk. Eyes with congenital conditions with retinal degeneration, such as Marfan syndrome, should undergo proper preoperative retinal screening, and any predisposing conditions, such as lattice or holes, should be lasered. There was no retinal detachment reported in our 1-year results, our pediatric glued IOLs, or case series with foldable glued IOL.[3,6,24] However, in the review of 486 eyes series with a rigid PMMA IOL, a late retinal detachment rate of 1% was reported.[9]

Hypotony

IOP less than 5 mm Hg is considered hypotony. Improper or inadequate intraoperative fluid maintenance can occasionally lead to postoperative hypotony. Wound leak and choroidal detachments should be excluded in the postoperative period, especially in eyes with a rigid IOL and trauma. The use of an AC maintainer or trocar infusion through the pars plana is vital for maintaining chamber pressure.[4,5] McKee et al[27] noted that self-resolving hypotony occurred in 11 (22%) eyes.

Pigment Dispersion and Iris Changes

These complications are often seen in eyes with predisposing conditions such as uveitis, trauma, or pigment dispersion syndrome. In our long-term study, 9 (15%) of 60 eyes had pigment dispersion on the IOL surface, which was seen as hyperreflective spots on the optic.[15] Of 9 eyes with pigment dispersion, 6 had a rigid IOL and 3 had a foldable IOL implanted. Iris adhesion to the optic was seen in 4 (6.6%) eyes, and optic capture was seen in 2, which resolved after dilation with tropicamide.

CONCLUSION

IOL implantation in eyes that lack PC support can be very challenging. Various techniques have been developed to provide IOL fixation in these cases with transscleral fixation. Managing complications with ease is the main objective of any new technique. The glued IOL procedure has shown satisfactory results. We aim to make the technique simpler and more refined for all complicated eyes, so that there would not be any clinical condition that hinders IOL implantation. We believe that glued IOL surgery is a good alternative in cases of inadequate capsular support.

REFERENCES

1. Agarwal A, Kumar DA, Jacob S, et al. Fibrin glue-assisted sutureless posterior chamber intraocular lens implantation in eyes with deficient posterior capsules. *J Cataract Refract Surg.* 2008;34(9):1433-1438.
2. Agarwal A, Kumar DA, Prakash G, et al. Fibrin glue-assisted sutureless posterior chamber intraocular lens implantation in eyes with deficient posterior capsules [reply to letter]. *J Cataract Refract Surg.* 2009;35(5):795-796.
3. Kumar DA, Agarwal A, Prakash G, et al. Glued posterior chamber IOL in eyes with deficient capsular support: a retrospective analysis of 1-year postoperative outcomes. *Eye (Lond).* 2010;24:1143-1148.
4. Kumar DA, Agarwal A, Agarwal A, et al. Glued intraocular lens implantation for eyes with defective capsules: a retrospective analysis of anatomical and functional outcome. *Saudi J Ophthalmol.* 2011;25(3):245-254.
5. Kumar DA, Agarwal A, Jacob S, et al. Use of 23-gauge or 25-gauge trocar cannula for globe maintenance in glued intraocular lens surgery. *J Cataract Refract Surg.* 2010;36(4):690-691.
6. Kumar DA, Agarwal A, Prakash D, et al. Glued intrascleral fixation of posterior chamber intraocular lens in children. *Am J Ophthalmol.* 2012;153(4):594-601.
7. Prakash G, Agarwal A, Kumar DA, et al. Translocation of malpositioned posterior chamber intraocular lens from anterior to posterior chamber along with fibrin glue-assisted transscleral fixation. *Eye Contact Lens.* 2010;36(1):45-48.

8. Agarwal A, Jacob S, Kumar DA, Agarwal A, Narasimhan S, Agarwal A. Handshake technique for glued intrascleral haptic fixation of a posterior chamber intraocular lens. *J Cataract Refract Surg.* 2013;39(3):317-322.
9. Kumar DA, Agarwal A. Glued intraocular lens: a major review on surgical technique and results. *Curr Opin Ophthalmol.* 2013;24:21-29.
10. Kumar DA, Agarwal A, Jacob S, Lamba M, Packialakshmi S, Meduri A. Combined surgical management of capsular and iris deficiency with glued intraocular lens technique. *J Refract Surg.* 2013;29:342-347.
11. Sinha R, Bali SJ, Sharma N, Titiyal JS. Fibrin glue-assisted fixation of decentered posterior chamber intraocular lens. *Eye Contact Lens.* 2012;38(1):68-71.
12. Ganekal S, Venkataratnam S, Dorairaj S, Jhanji V. Comparative evaluation of suture-assisted and fibrin glue-assisted scleral fixated intraocular lens implantation. *J Refract Surg.* 2012;28(4):249-252.
13. Kumar DA, Agarwal A, Jacob S, et al. Repositioning of the dislocated intraocular lens with sutureless 20-gauge vitrectomy retina. *Retina.* 2010;30(4):682-687.
14. Kumar DA, Agarwal A, Prakash G, Jacob S. Managing total aniridia with aphakia using a glued iris prosthesis. *J Cataract Refract Surg.* 2010;36(5):864-865.
15. Kumar DA, Agarwal A, Agarwal A, Chandrasekar R, Priyanka V. Long-term assessment of tilt of glued intraocular lenses: an optical coherence tomography analysis 5 years after surgery. *Ophthalmology.* 2015;122(1):48-55.
16. Kumar DA, Agarwal A, Jacob S, Agarwal A. Glued transscleral intraocular lens exchange for anterior chamber lenses in complicated eyes: analysis of indications and results. Am J Ophthalmol. 2013;156(6):1125-1133.
17. Prakash G, Jacob S, Kumar DA, et al. Femtosecond assisted keratoplasty with fibrin glue assisted sutureless posterior chamber lens implantation: a new triple procedure. *J Cataract Refract Surg.* 2009;35(6):973-979.
18. Prakash G, Agarwal A, Jacob S, et al. Femtosecond-assisted Descemet stripping automated endothelial keratoplasty with fibrin glue-assisted sutureless posterior chamber lens implantation. *Cornea.* 2010;29(11):1315-1319.
19. Sinha R, Shekhar H, Sharma N, et al. Intrascleral fibrin glue intraocular lens fixation combined with Descemet-stripping automated endothelial keratoplasty or penetrating keratoplasty. *J Cataract Refract Surg.* 2012;38(7):1240-1245.
20. Nair V, Kumar DA, Prakash G, et al. Bilateral spontaneous in-the-bag anterior subluxation of PC IOL managed with glued IOL technique: a case report. *Eye Contact Lens.* 2009;35(4):215-217.
21. Kumar DA, Agarwal A, Gabor SG, et al. Sutureless sclera fixated posterior chamber intraocular lens [Letter to editor]. *J Cataract Refract Surg.* 2011;37:2089-2090.
22. Gabor SG, Pavilidis MM. Sutureless intrascleral posterior chamber intraocular lens fixation. *J Cataract Refract Surg.* 2007;33(11):1851-1854.
23. Maggi R, Maggi C. Sutureless scleral fixation of intraocular lenses. *J Cataract Refract Surg.* 1997;23(9):1289-1294.
24. Kumar DA, Agarwal A, Packiyalakshmi S, Jacob S, Agarwal A. Complications and visual outcomes after glued foldable intraocular lens implantation in eyes with inadequate capsules. *J Cataract Refract Surg.* 2013;39(8):1211-1218.
25. Ashok Kumar D, Agarwal A, Agarwal A, Chandrasekar R. Clinical outcomes of glued transscleral fixated intraocular lens in functionally one-eyed patients. *Eye Contact Lens.* 2014;40(4):e23-e28.
26. Kumar DA, Agarwal A, Packiyalakshmi S, Agarwal A. In vivo analysis of glued intraocular lens position with ultrasound biomicroscopy. *J Cataract Refract Surg.* 2013;39(7):1017-1022.

27. McKee Y, Price FW Jr, Feng MT, Price MO. Implementation of the posterior chamber intraocular lens intrascleral haptic fixation technique (glued intraocular lens) in a United States practice: outcomes and insights. *J Cataract Refract Surg.* 2014;40(12):2099-2105.

28. Narang P, Narang S. Glue-assisted intrascleral fixation of posterior chamber intraocular lens. *Indian J Ophthalmol.* 2013;61(4):163-167.

29. Jacob S, Agarwal A, Agarwal A, Narasimhan S. Closed-chamber haptic reexternalization for posteriorly displaced sclerotomy and inadequate haptic tuck in glued posterior chamber intraocular lenses. *J Cataract Refract Surg.* 2015;41(2):268-271.

30. Narang P. Complications of glued IOL. In: *Glued IOL.* Jaypee Publishers; 2012.

31. Beiko G, Steinert R. Modification of externalized haptic support of glued intraocular lens technique. *J Cataract Refract Surg.* 2013;39(3):323-325.

32. Loya N, Lichter H, Barash D, Goldenberg-Cohen N, Strassmann E, Weinberger D. Posterior chamber intraocular lens implantation after capsular tear: ultrasound biomicroscopy evaluation. *J Cataract Refract Surg.* 2001;27(9):1423-1427.

33. Sewelam A, Ismail AM, El Serogy H. Ultrasound biomicroscopy of haptic position after transscleral fixation of posterior chamber intraocular lenses. *J Cataract Refract Surg.* 2001;27(9):1418-1422.

34. Ashok Kumar D, Agarwal A, Sivangnanam S, Chandrasekar R, Agarwal A. Implantation of glued intraocular lenses in eyes with microcornea. *J Cataract Refract Surg.* 2015;41(2):327-333.

35. Agarwal A, Narang P, Kumar D, Agarwal A. Clinical outcomes of sleeveless phacotip assisted levitation of dropped nucleus. *Br J Ophthalmol.* 2014;98(10):1429-1434.

36. Lee SJ, Kim IG, Park JM. Management of posteriorly dislocated crystalline lens with perfluorocarbon liquid and fibrin glue-assisted scleral-fixated intraocular lens implantation. *J Cataract Refract Surg.* 2013;39(3):334-338.

37. Agarwal A, Kumar DA, Nair V. Cataract surgery in the setting of trauma. *Curr Opin Ophthalmol.* 2010;21(1):65-70.

38. Prakash G, Ashokumar D, Jacob S, Kumar KS, Agarwal A, Agarwal A. Anterior segment optical coherence tomography-aided diagnosis and primary posterior chamber intraocular lens implantation with fibrin glue in traumatic phacocele with scleral perforation. *J Cataract Refract Surg.* 2009;35(4):782-784.

Financial Disclosures

Dr. Amar Agarwal is a consultant for Abbott Medical Optics, STAAR Surgical Company, and Bausch + Lomb.

Ashvin Agarwal has no financial or proprietary interest in the materials presented herein.

Dr. Athiya Agarwal has no financial or proprietary interest in the materials presented herein.

Dr. Soosan Jacob has no financial or proprietary interest in the materials presented herein.

Dr. Vishal Jhanjhi has no financial or proprietary interest in the materials presented herein.

Dr. Dhivya Ashok Kumar has no financial or proprietary interest in the materials presented herein.

Priya Narang has no financial or proprietary interest in the materials presented herein.

Index

Printed in the United States
by Baker & Taylor Publisher Services